Obesity

Editor: Danielle Lobban

Volume 436

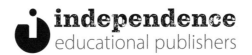
independence
educational publishers

First published by Independence Educational Publishers

The Studio, High Green

Great Shelford

Cambridge CB22 5EG

England

© Independence 2024

ISBN-13: 978 1 86168 896 5

Printed in Great Britain

Zenith Print Group

Acknowledgements

The publisher is grateful for permission to reproduce the material in this book. While every care has been taken to trace and acknowledge copyright, the publisher tenders its apology for any accidental infringement or where copyright has proved untraceable. The publisher would be pleased to come to a suitable arrangement in any such case with the rightful owner.

The material reproduced in **issues** books is provided as an educational resource only. The views, opinions and information contained within reprinted material in **issues** books do not necessarily represent those of Independence Educational Publishers and its employees.

Images

Cover image courtesy of iStock. All other images courtesy of Freepik, Pixabay and Unsplash.

Additional acknowledgements

With thanks to the Independence team: Shelley Baldry, Tracy Biram, Klaudia Sommer and Jackie Staines.

Danielle Lobban

Cambridge, January 2024

Contents

Introduction

Obesity is Volume 436 in the **issues** series. The aim of the series is to offer current, diverse information about important issues in our world, from a UK perspective.

About Obesity

In the UK around 1 in 4 adults are obese. This book explores the problem with obesity, what causes obesity, how it can affect your health, and how to maintain a healthy weight.

Our sources

Titles in the **issues** series are designed to function as educational resource books, providing a balanced overview of a specific subject.

The information in our books is comprised of facts, articles and opinions from many different sources, including:

- Newspaper reports and opinion pieces
- Website factsheets
- Magazine and journal articles
- Statistics and surveys
- Government reports
- Literature from special interest groups.

A note on critical evaluation

Because the information reprinted here is from a number of different sources, readers should bear in mind the origin of the text and whether the source is likely to have a particular bias when presenting information (or when conducting their research). It is hoped that, as you read about the many aspects of the issues explored in this book, you will critically evaluate the information presented.

It is important that you decide whether you are being presented with facts or opinions. Does the writer give a biased or unbiased report? If an opinion is being expressed, do you agree with the writer? Is there potential bias to the 'facts' or statistics behind an article?

Activities

Throughout this book, you will find a selection of assignments and activities designed to help you engage with the articles you have been reading and to explore your own opinions. Some tasks will take longer than others and there is a mixture of design, writing and research-based activities that you can complete alone or in a group.

Further research

At the end of each article we have listed its source and a website that you can visit if you would like to conduct your own research. Please remember to critically evaluate any sources that you consult and consider whether the information you are viewing is accurate and unbiased.

Issues Online

The **issues** series of books is complemented by our online resource, issuesonline.co.uk

On the Issues Online website you will find a wealth of information, covering over 70 topics, to support the PSHE and RSE curriculum.

Why Issues Online?

Researching a topic? Issues Online is the best place to start for...

Librarians

Issues Online is an essential tool for librarians: feel confident you are signposting safe, reliable, user-friendly online resources to students and teaching staff alike. We provide multi-user concurrent access, so no waiting around for another student to finish with a resource. Issues Online also provides FREE downloadable posters for your shelf/wall/table displays.

Teachers

Issues Online is an ideal resource for lesson planning, inspiring lively debate in class and setting lessons and homework tasks.

Our accessible, engaging content helps deepen students' knowledge, promotes critical thinking and develops independent learning skills.

Issues Online saves precious preparation time. We wade through the wealth of material on the internet to filter the best quality, most relevant and up-to-date information you need to start exploring a topic.

Our carefully selected, balanced content presents an overview and insight into each topic from a variety of sources and viewpoints.

Students

Issues Online is designed to support your studies in a broad range of topics, particularly social issues relevant to young people today.

Thousands of articles, statistics and infographs instantly available to help you with research and assignments.

With 24/7 access using the powerful Algolia search system, you can find relevant information quickly, easily and safely anytime from your laptop, tablet or smartphone, in class or at home.

Visit issuesonline.co.uk to find out more!

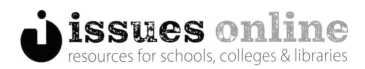

What is obesity?

According to the World Obesity Federation; *'Obesity is a medical condition described as excess body weight in the form of fat. When accumulated, this fat can lead to severe health impairments.'*

Commonly, Body Mass Index, which takes into account your height and weight, is used to determine if someone is a healthy weight. For most adults, a BMI of:

* 18.5 to 24.9 - healthy weight

* 25 to 29.9 - overweight

* 30 to 39.9 - obesity

* 40 or above - severe obesity

However, BMI is a very crude measure, and is not used on its own to diagnose obesity. Other factors, such as your gender, ethnicity, body composition and age should be taken into account. You can use the NHS BMI calculator to check yours.

Other measures, such as waist circumference, can be used to diagnose whether someone is living with obesity and to assess their risk of developing other health conditions such as Type 2 diabetes.

What causes obesity?

Obesity is a complex condition influenced by many factors. These include diet, activity levels, genetics (your DNA), other diseases or conditions, medications, mental health, sleep, weight stigma, poverty or your environment. In most cases it will be a combination of many these factors and is not simply driven by eating too much and not enough exercise.

Critically, it is important not to just think of obesity as an issue of personal responsibility or failure. Helping the population to reach and maintain a healthy weight will require lots of different policy changes – there is no one solution that will have enough impact, it requires the whole system to change.

What is the best way to lose weight?

There is no one best way to lose weight, which is why dietitians work to understand your personal circumstances when making recommendations. Improving your diet and increasing activity can be key to losing weight, although are not the only factors that need to be considered.

When aiming to lose weight it is important to have realistic goals that are achievable. Success boosts confidence in your ability to lose weight. A weight loss of between 0.5 to 2 pounds (0.5-1kg) a week is a safe and realistic target.

There is no quick fix. People who successfully lose weight and keep it off develop techniques to make their new lifestyle and activity habits an enjoyable way of life and also make them life long.

What is weight stigma?

Weight stigma, also known as weight bias, is the discrimination or stereotyping of a person based on their weight or body size.

Weight stigma can be damaging to mental health, increase metabolic risk factors and further reducing self-esteem. Weight stigma is unhelpful in supporting people to better manage their weight and has been shown in in fact result in increased calorie intake and increased body weight over time.

How do dietitians support people living with obesity?

Obesity specialist dietitians work with adults and children, alongside their families, to form a plan for eating patterns, food, activity levels and wellbeing that takes into account personal goals, preferences and cultural needs. They often work with other healthcare professionals such as doctors, physiotherapists and psychologists. Other obesity dietitians research obesity and its treatment, or work in public health to provide population level advice to help people reach or maintain a healthy weight.

What are the 'tiers' or 'levels' of weight management?

This definition is adapted from National Institute of Health and Care Excellence (NICE).

Different tiers or levels of weight management services cover different activities. Definitions vary locally but usually;

* Tier 1 covers universal services (such as health promotion, public health services or primary care)

* Tier 2 covers lifestyle interventions such as commercial weight loss programmes or seeing your GP or nurse for advice.

* Tier 3 covers specialist weight management services for those that need more specialist support.

* Tier 4 covers weight loss (bariatric) surgery.

The above information is reprinted with kind permission from The British Dietetic Association

© 2023 British Dietetic Association

www.bda.uk.com

Obesity and overweight

What are obesity and overweight?

Overweight and obesity are defined as abnormal or excessive fat accumulation that may impair health.

Body mass index (BMI) is a simple index of weight-for-height that is commonly used to classify overweight and obesity in adults. It is defined as a person's weight in kilograms divided by the square of his height in meters (kg/m2).

Adults

For adults, WHO defines overweight and obesity as follows:

- overweight is a BMI greater than or equal to 25; and

- obesity is a BMI greater than or equal to 30.

BMI provides the most useful population-level measure of overweight and obesity as it is the same for both sexes and for all ages of adults. However, it should be considered a rough guide because it may not correspond to the same degree of fatness in different individuals.

For children, age needs to be considered when defining overweight and obesity.

Children under 5 years of age

For children under 5 years of age:

- overweight is weight-for-height greater than 2 standard deviations above WHO Child Growth Standards median; and

- obesity is weight-for-height greater than 3 standard deviations above the WHO Child Growth Standards median.

Children aged between 5–19 years

Overweight and obesity are defined as follows for children aged between 5–19 years:

- overweight is BMI-for-age greater than 1 standard deviation above the WHO Growth Reference median; and

- obesity is greater than 2 standard deviations above the WHO Growth Reference median.

Facts about overweight and obesity

Some recent WHO global estimates follow.

- In 2016, more than 1.9 billion adults aged 18 years and older were overweight. Of these over 650 million adults were obese.

- In 2016, 39% of adults aged 18 years and over (39% of men and 40% of women) were overweight.

- Overall, about 13% of the world's adult population (11% of men and 15% of women) were obese in 2016.

- The worldwide prevalence of obesity nearly tripled between 1975 and 2016.

In 2019, an estimated 38.2 million children under the age of 5 years were overweight or obese. Once considered a high-income country problem, overweight and obesity are now on the rise in low- and middle-income countries, particularly in urban settings. In Africa, the number of overweight children under 5 has increased by nearly 24% percent since 2000. Almost half of the children under 5 who were overweight or obese in 2019 lived in Asia.

Over 340 million children and adolescents aged 5–19 were overweight or obese in 2016.

The prevalence of overweight and obesity among children and adolescents aged 5–19 has risen dramatically from just 4% in 1975 to just over 18% in 2016. The rise has occurred similarly among both boys and girls: in 2016 18% of girls and 19% of boys were overweight.

While just under 1% of children and adolescents aged 5-19 were obese in 1975, more than 124 million children and adolescents (6% of girls and 8% of boys) were obese in 2016.

Overweight and obesity are linked to more deaths worldwide than underweight. Globally there are more people who are obese than underweight – this occurs in every region except parts of sub-Saharan Africa and Asia.

What causes obesity and overweight?

The fundamental cause of obesity and overweight is an energy imbalance between calories consumed and calories expended. Globally, there has been:

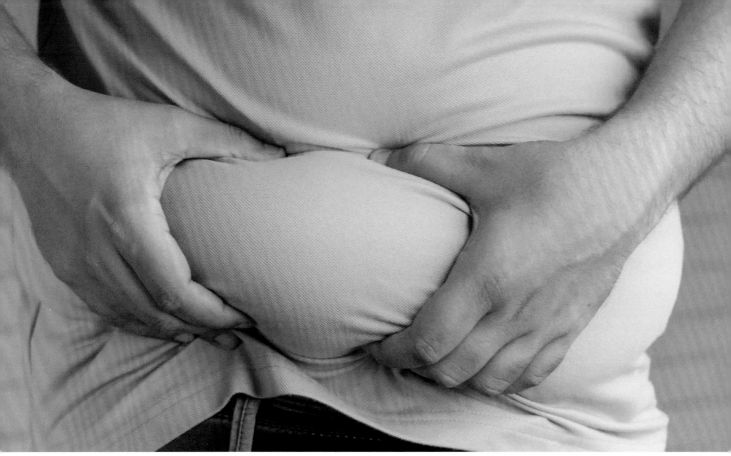

- an increased intake of energy-dense foods that are high in fat and sugars; and

- an increase in physical inactivity due to the increasingly sedentary nature of many forms of work, changing modes of transportation, and increasing urbanization.

Changes in dietary and physical activity patterns are often the result of environmental and societal changes associated with development and lack of supportive policies in sectors such as health, agriculture, transport, urban planning, environment, food processing, distribution, marketing, and education.

What are common health consequences of overweight and obesity?

Raised BMI is a major risk factor for noncommunicable diseases such as:

- cardiovascular diseases (mainly heart disease and stroke), which were the leading cause of death in 2012;

- diabetes;

- musculoskeletal disorders (especially osteoarthritis – a highly disabling degenerative disease of the joints);

- some cancers (including endometrial, breast, ovarian, prostate, liver, gallbladder, kidney, and colon).

The risk for these noncommunicable diseases increases with increases in BMI.

Childhood obesity is associated with a higher chance of obesity, premature death and disability in adulthood. But in addition to increased future risks, obese children experience breathing difficulties, increased risk of fractures, hypertension, early markers of cardiovascular disease, insulin resistance and psychological effects.

Facing a double burden of malnutrition

Many low- and middle-income countries are now facing a 'double burden' of malnutrition.

- While these countries continue to deal with the problems of infectious diseases and undernutrition, they are also experiencing a rapid upsurge in noncommunicable disease risk factors such as obesity and overweight, particularly in urban settings.

- It is not uncommon to find undernutrition and obesity co-existing within the same country, the same community and the same household.

Children in low- and middle-income countries are more vulnerable to inadequate pre-natal, infant, and young child nutrition. At the same time, these children are exposed to high-fat, high-sugar, high-salt, energy-dense, and micronutrient-poor foods, which tend to be lower in cost but also lower in nutrient quality. These dietary patterns, in conjunction with lower levels of physical activity, result in sharp increases in childhood obesity while undernutrition issues remain unsolved.

How can overweight and obesity be reduced?

Overweight and obesity, as well as their related noncommunicable diseases, are largely preventable. Supportive environments and communities are fundamental in shaping people's choices, by making the choice of healthier foods and regular physical activity the easiest

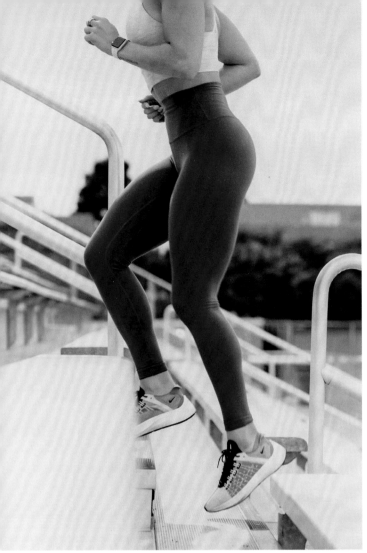

choice (the choice that is the most accessible, available and affordable), and therefore preventing overweight and obesity.

At the individual level, people can:

- limit energy intake from total fats and sugars;

- increase consumption of fruit and vegetables, as well as legumes, whole grains and nuts; and

- engage in regular physical activity (60 minutes a day for children and 150 minutes spread through the week for adults).

Individual responsibility can only have its full effect where people have access to a healthy lifestyle. Therefore, at the societal level it is important to support individuals in following the recommendations above, through sustained implementation of evidence based and population based policies that make regular physical activity and healthier dietary choices available, affordable and easily accessible to everyone, particularly to the poorest individuals. An example of such a policy is a tax on sugar sweetened beverages.

The food industry can play a significant role in promoting healthy diets by:

- reducing the fat, sugar and salt content of processed foods;

- ensuring that healthy and nutritious choices are available and affordable to all consumers;

- restricting marketing of foods high in sugars, salt and fats, especially those foods aimed at children and teenagers; and

- ensuring the availability of healthy food choices and supporting regular physical activity practice in the workplace.

WHO response

Adopted by the World Health Assembly in 2004 and recognized again in a 2011 political declaration on noncommunicable disease (NCDs), the 'WHO Global Strategy on Diet, Physical Activity and Health' describes the actions needed to support healthy diets and regular physical activity. The Strategy calls upon all stakeholders to take action at global, regional and local levels to improve diets and physical activity patterns at the population level.

The 2030 Agenda for Sustainable Development recognizes NCDs as a major challenge for sustainable development. As part of the Agenda, Heads of State and Government committed to develop ambitious national responses, by 2030, to reduce by one-third premature mortality from NCDs through prevention and treatment (SDG target 3.4).

The 'Global action plan on physical activity 2018–2030: more active people for a healthier world' provides effective and feasible policy actions to increase physical activity globally. WHO published ACTIVE, a technical package to assist countries in planning and delivery of their responses. New WHO guidelines on physical activity, sedentary behavior and sleep in children under five years of age were launched in 2019.

The World Health Assembly welcomed the report of the Commission on Ending Childhood Obesity (2016) and its 6 recommendations to address the obesogenic environment and critical periods in the life course to tackle childhood obesity. The implementation plan to guide countries in taking action to implement the recommendations of the Commission was welcomed by the World Health Assembly in 2017.

9 June 2021

What is the body mass index (BMI)?

The body mass index (BMI) is a measure that uses your height and weight to work out if your weight is healthy.

The BMI calculation divides an adult's weight in kilograms by their height in metres squared. For example, A BMI of 25 means 25kg/m2.

BMI ranges

For most adults, an ideal BMI is in the 18.5 to 24.9 range.

For children and young people aged 2 to 18, the BMI calculation takes into account age and gender as well as height and weight.

If your BMI is:

* below 18.5 – you're in the underweight range
* between 18.5 and 24.9 – you're in the healthy weight range
* between 25 and 29.9 – you're in the overweight range
* 30 or over – you're in the obese range

If you want to calculate your BMI, you can use the healthy weight calculator on the NHS website.

Accuracy of BMI

BMI takes into account natural variations in body shape, giving a healthy weight range for a particular height.

As well as measuring your BMI, healthcare professionals may take other factors into account when assessing if you're a healthy weight.

Muscle is much denser than fat, so very muscular people, such as heavyweight boxers, weight trainers and athletes, may be a healthy weight even though their BMI is classed as obese.

Your ethnic group can also affect your risk of some health conditions. For example, adults of South Asian origin may have a higher risk of some health problems, such as diabetes, with a BMI of 23, which is usually considered healthy.

You should not use BMI as a measure if you're pregnant. Get advice from your midwife or GP if you're concerned about your weight.

28 November 2022

Body Mass Index
(BMI)

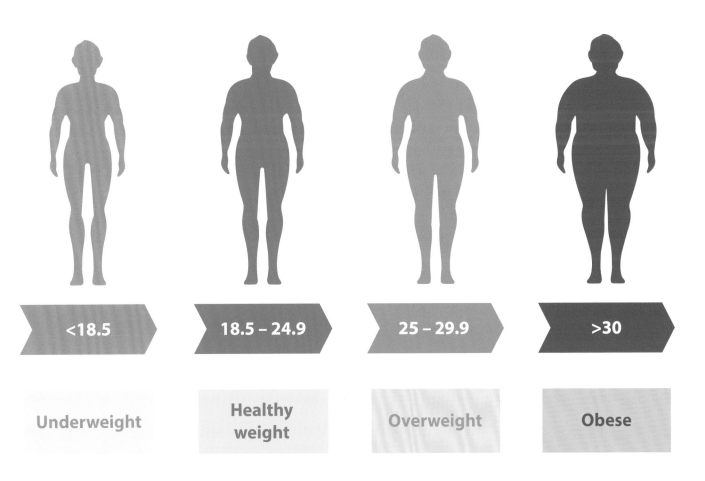

<18.5	18.5 – 24.9	25 – 29.9	>30
Underweight	Healthy weight	Overweight	Obese

Causes of obesity

Obesity is a complex issue with many causes. It's caused when extra calories are stored in the body as fat.

If you consume high amounts of energy, particularly found in high fat and high sugar foods, and do not use all of the energy through physical activity, much of the extra energy will be stored in the body as fat.

Calories

The energy value of food is measured in units called calories. The average physically active man needs about 2,500 calories a day to maintain a healthy weight, and the average physically active woman needs about 2,000 calories a day.

This amount of calories may sound high, but it can be easy to reach if you eat certain types of food. For example, eating a large takeaway hamburger, fries and a milkshake can total 1,500 calories – and that's just 1 meal. For more information, read our guide to understanding calories.

As well as this, many people do not meet the recommended physical activity levels for adults, so excess calories consumed end up being stored as fat in the body.

Diet

Diet and lifestyle factors contribute to development of obesity and overweight. Some of the most common ones are:

- eating large amounts of processed or fast food – this is food that's high in fat and sugar
- drinking too much alcohol – alcohol contains a lot of calories
- eating out a lot – food cooked in a restaurant may be higher in fat and sugar
- eating larger portions than you need
- drinking too many sugary drinks – including soft drinks and fruit juice
- comfort eating – some people may comfort eat due to many other factors affecting their life such as low self-esteem or low mood

Changes in society have also made it more difficult to have a healthy diet. High calorie food has become cheaper and more convenient, and is heavily advertised and promoted.

Physical activity

Lack of physical activity is another important factor related to obesity. Many people have jobs that involve sitting at a desk for most of the day. They also rely on their cars, rather than walking or cycling.

For relaxation, many people tend to watch TV, browse the internet or play computer games, and rarely take regular exercise.

If you are not active enough, you do not use the energy provided by the food you eat, and the extra energy you consume is stored by the body as fat.

The Department of Health and Social Care recommends that adults do at least 150 minutes of moderate-intensity aerobic activity, such as cycling or fast walking, every week. This does not need to be done all in a single session, but can be broken down into smaller periods. For example, you could exercise for 30 minutes a day for 5 days a week.

If you're living with obesity and trying to lose weight, you may need to do more exercise than this. It may help to start off slowly and gradually increase the amount of exercise you do each week.

Genetics

There are some genes associated with obesity and overweight. In some people, genes can affect how their bodies change food into energy and store fat. Genes can also affect people's lifestyle choices.

There are also some rare genetic conditions that can cause obesity, such as Prader-Willi syndrome.

Certain genetic traits inherited from your parents – such as having a large appetite – may make losing weight more difficult, but they do not make it impossible.

In many cases, obesity is more to do with environmental factors, such as not having easy access to healthy food, or unhealthy eating habits learned during childhood.

Medical reasons

In some cases, underlying medical conditions may contribute to weight gain. These include:

- an underactive thyroid gland (hypothyroidism) – where your thyroid gland does not produce enough hormones
- Cushing's syndrome – a rare disorder that causes the over-production of steroid hormones

However, if conditions such as these are properly diagnosed and treated, they should pose less of a barrier to weight loss.

Certain medicines, including some steroids, medications for epilepsy and diabetes, and some medications used to treat mental illness – including some antidepressants and medicines for schizophrenia – can contribute to weight gain.

Weight gain can sometimes be a side effect of stopping smoking.

15 February 2023

Obesity statistics

An extract.

By Carl Baker

Obesity in England: summary

In England, men are more likely to have a body mass index measurement above normal than women.

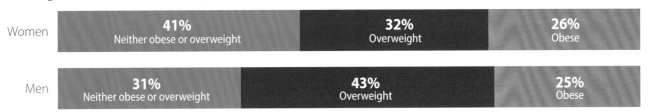

| Women | 41% Neither obese or overweight | 32% Overweight | 26% Obese |
| Men | 31% Neither obese or overweight | 43% Overweight | 25% Obese |

Around three quarters of those aged 45-74 are overweight or obese.

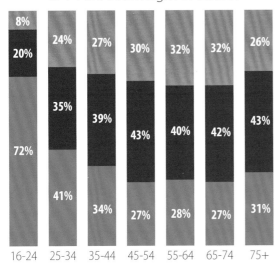

	16-24	25-34	35-44	45-54	55-64	65-74	75+
	8%	24%	27%	30%	32%	32%	26%
	20%	35%	39%	43%	40%	42%	43%
	72%	41%	34%	27%	28%	27%	31%

Obesity levels increased from 15% in 1993 to 28% in 2019.

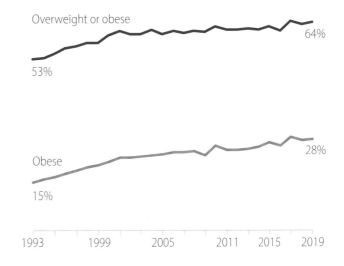

Overweight or obese
53% ... 64%

Obese
15% ... 28%

1993   1999   2005   2011   2015   2019

One in ten children is obese by age 5, rising to 23% by age 11.

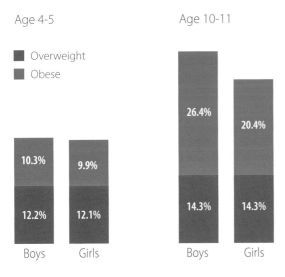

Age 4-5   Age 10-11

- ■ Overweight
- ■ Obese

	Boys	Girls
Age 4-5 Obese	10.3%	9.9%
Age 4-5 Overweight	12.2%	12.1%
Age 10-11 Obese	26.4%	20.4%
Age 10-11 Overweight	14.3%	14.3%

Deprived children are more likely to be obese, and the gap has widened.

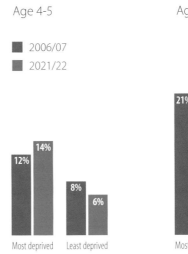
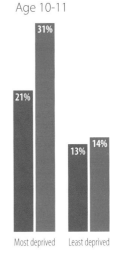

Age 4-5   Age 10-11

- ■ 2006/07
- ■ 2021/22

Age 4-5 — Most deprived: 12%, 14%. Least deprived: 8%, 6%.

Age 10-11 — Most deprived: 21%, 31%. Least deprived: 13%, 14%.

Source: Obesity Statistics, House of Commons Library

Obesity among adults in England

The Health Survey for England, published by NHS Digital, provides estimates of obesity levels based on the body mass index (BMI) of a representative sample of people aged 16+. The 2021 survey was based on adjusted self- reported height and weight data, while in previous years the survey was based on measured data.1

In the 2021 survey, 25.9% of adults in England were obese and a further 37.9% were overweight, making a total of 63.8% who were either overweight or obese. Men were more likely than women to be overweight or obese.

Out of every 1,000 adults in England...

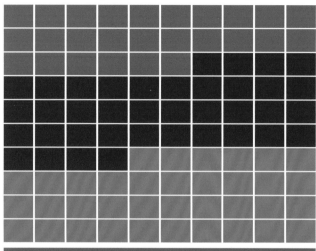

259 are obese

379 are overweight

362 are neither overweight or obese

Source: NHS Digital, Health Survey for England 2021, Table 1

Obesity among children in England

The National Child Measurement Programme (NCMP) found in 2021/22 that 10.1% of reception age children in England (ages 4-5) were obese, with a further 12.1% overweight. These proportions were higher among year 6 children (age 10-11), with 23.4% being obese and 14.3% overweight.

The 2020/21 edition of the survey, which was carried out as a sample because of the Covid-19 pandemic, found large increases compared to previous years, with obesity levels at 14.4% in reception and 25.5% in year 6.

In the 2021/22 survey prevalence was lower, but the figures were still higher than in previous years.

In both age groups, boys are slightly more likely than girls to be obese. This difference is less than one percentage point at ages 4-5 but rises to six percentage points among ages 10-11.

Childhood obesity and deprivation

Children living in more deprived areas are substantially more likely to be obese. In 2021/22, 6.2% of children aged 4-5 living in the least deprived tenth of areas of England were obese. This compares with 13.6% of those living in the most deprived tenth of areas.

Of every 1,000 10 & 11 year olds in England...

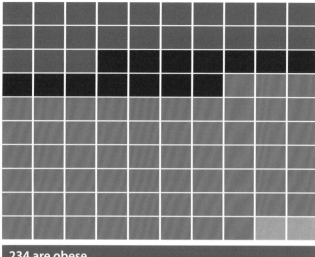

234 are obese

143 are overweight

608 are of healthy weight

15 are underweight

Of every 1,000 4 & 5 year olds in England...

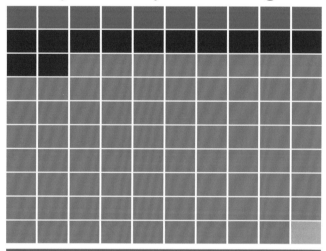

101 are obese

121 are overweight

765 are of healthy weight

12 are underweight

Source: NHS Digital, National Child Measurement Programme 2021/22, Table 1a

In Year 6 (ages 10-11), 13.5% of children living in the least deprived areas were obese, compared with 31.3% in the most deprived areas. In both age groups, children in the most deprived areas were approximately twice as likely to be obese. Rates of severe obesity were around four times higher in the most deprived areas.

Scotland: adult obesity

Adult obesity in Scotland is recorded as part of the Scottish Health Survey, published by the Scottish Government. In 2021, figures were based on adjusted self-reported height and weight measures. 31% of adults were obese (BMI over 30) and a further 36% were overweight (BMI between 25 and 30).

Measures of obesity and excess weight

The most widely used measure of obesity is the Body Mass Index (BMI), defined as weight divided by the square of height (kg/m2). A person is classified as 'obese' if their BMI is 30 or higher, and 'overweight' if their BMI is between 25 and 30. A BMI of 40 or more is often known as 'morbid obesity'. 'Excess weight' is an umbrella term for BMI over 25, ie either overweight or obese.

BMI is not always definitive and may not be appropriate for all groups, and sometimes other measures are used. These include waist circumference and the waist-hip ratio.

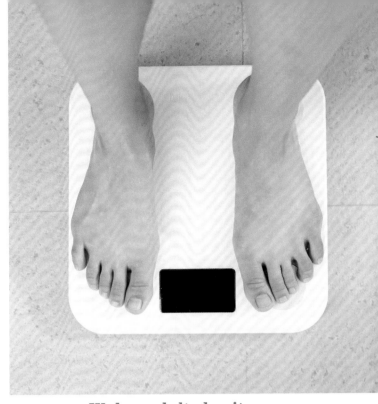

A higher proportion of men than women were overweight, but a higher proportion of women than men were obese. In all age groups over 55, more than 70% of people were overweight or obese.

Scotland: child obesity

The Scottish Health Survey also contains information on BMI for children.

The 2021 survey found that 20% of children aged 2-6 were obese, 22% of children aged 7-11, and rising again to 12% of children aged 12-15. Overall, boys were more likely (20%) than girls (16%) to be obese.

Obesity was more common in children living in households with lower incomes.

Child obesity in this survey is classified as those who are above the 95th percentile of the 1990 UK growth reference standards.

Wales: adult obesity

Adult obesity in Wales is recorded in the National Survey for Wales based on self-reported data.

In 2021/22, 26% of women and 23% of men reported being obese (BMI over 30). 67% of men were overweight or obese, compared with 58% of women.

Obesity was highest in the 45-64 age group (29%) and lowest in those aged 16-24 and 75+ (16%).

69% of men and 65% of women in Scotland were overweight or obese in 2021

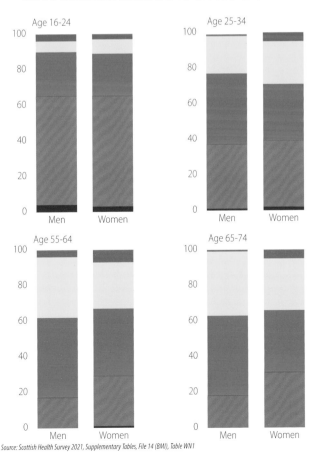

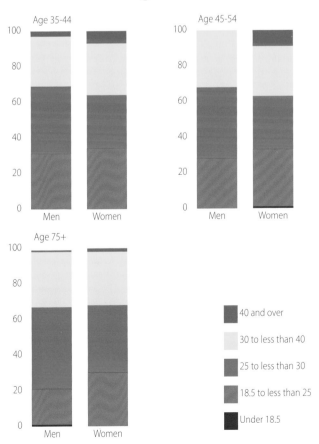

Legend:
- 40 and over
- 30 to less than 40
- 25 to less than 30
- 18.5 to less than 25
- Under 18.5

Source: Scottish Health Survey 2021, Supplementary Tables, File 14 (BMI), Table WN1

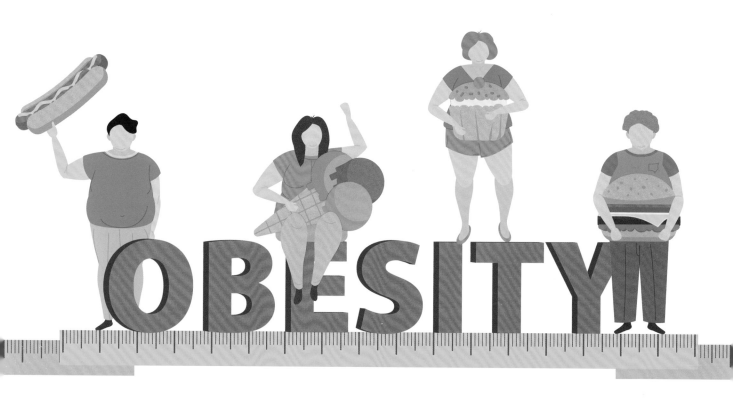

Wales: child obesity

The most recent comprehensive data on child obesity in Wales is from the 2018/19 Child Measurement Programme for Wales. Data collection for 2020/21 was interrupted by the Covid-19 pandemic, and data was only published for two health board areas.

In 2018/19, 12.6% of children aged 4-5 in Wales were obese and a further 14.4% were overweight. Children living in the most deprived areas of Wales were almost twice as likely to be obese (15.3%) as those in the least deprived areas (8.3%).

There were only small differences between obesity rates for boys and girls.

Obesity rates were estimated to be highest among children in Merthyr Tydfil and lowest in Monmouthshire and Vale of Glamorgan.

Northern Ireland: adult obesity

Data is available from the Health Survey Northern Ireland, but BMI questions were not asked in the two most recent editions.

In 2019/20, 27% of adults in Northern Ireland were obese, with a further 38% overweight. 71% of men were overweight or obese, compared with 60% of women. The chart below shows a breakdown by age.

Obesity levels in Northern Ireland are estimated to have increased from 23% in 2010/11 to 27% in 2019/20.

Of respondents who were overweight, 48% of women said they were trying to lose weight, compared with 24% of men.

In Northern Ireland, obesity rates are estimated to be highest among ages 65-74

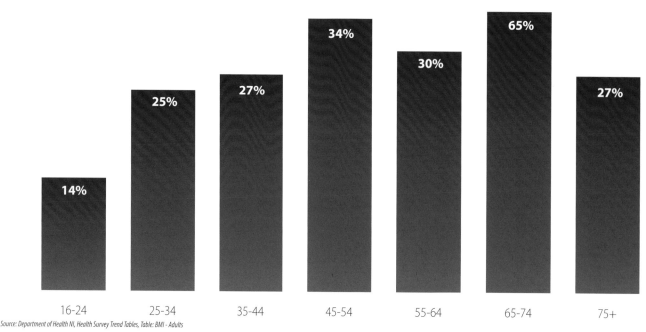

16-24	25-34	35-44	45-54	55-64	65-74	75+
14%	25%	27%	34%	30%	65%	27%

Source: Department of Health NI, Health Survey Trend Tables, Table: BMI - Adults

Obesity levels in countries with measured data

2020 or nearest year

Country	%		Country	%
United States	43%		Finland	27%
Mexico	36%		Canada	24%
Chile	34%		Germany	24%
Hungary	33%		Ireland	23%
Costa Rica	31%		Belgium	21%
New Zealand	31%		Czech Republic	21%
Australia	30%		Israel	19%
Türkiye	29%		France	16%
Portugal	29%		Korea	7%
UK	28%		Japan	5%

Source: OECD Health Statistics, Key Indicators file, Table: Obesity, total (M)

Northern Ireland: child obesity

In 2019/20, the Health Survey Northern Ireland recorded 7% of children aged 2-10 and 4% of children aged 11-15 as being obese. However, because of the survey's small sample size, meaningful comparisons over time or between age groups can't be made.

As mentioned above, this survey did not contain questions on BMI in the last two editions.

International comparisons

The OECD Health Statistics database collates data on obesity from different countries. The table above shows data for countries with measured (as opposed to self-reported) obesity monitoring, for 2020 or the most recent year available.

The United States had the highest measured percentage of people who were obese (43%), while the UK ranked tenth among these countries with 28%. Japan had the lowest measured obesity prevalence, at 5%.

12 January 2023

Tackling Obesity

The real reason we are getting fatter: experts say it's not as simple as overeating

Excess weight will soon overtake smoking as the number one cause of cancer, while type 2 diabetes is on the rise. But what exactly is behind our national weight issue?

By Sarah Graham

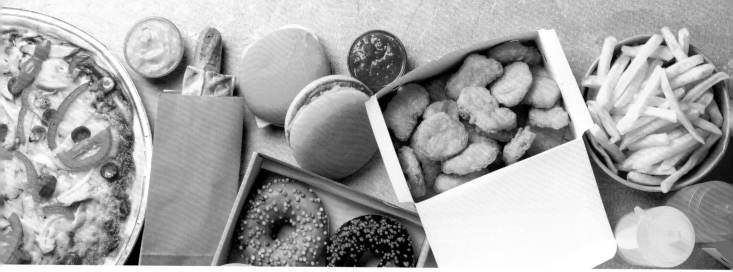

The proportion of adults in England who were classed as overweight or obese rose from 52.9 per cent in 1993 to 64.3 per cent in 2019, according to data from NHS Digital. But this isn't a trend born of only the last 30 years, the UK population has been seeing a steady increase in both its weight and size since the 50s and 60s, a shift which has been widely attributed to our changing lifestyles over the last half a century.

This change is already having an impact on our health with data published earlier in November showing that Type 2 diabetes is increasing at an 'alarming' rate among the under-40s. Cancer charities say that obesity is now the second biggest cause of the disease in the UK – with one in 20 cases caused by excess weight – and will overtake smoking to be the leading cause in the future. Such statistics have reignited longstanding concerns about the nation's expanding waistlines. But what exactly is behind our national weight issue?

'Historically our diet was focused on fuelling people to do manual labour for eight to 12 hours a day, whereas today many more of us are desk-based,' says Aisling Piggott, a registered dietician and spokesperson for the British Dietetic Association (BDA). As well as a change in working habits, and related activity levels, Ms Piggott says 'the British diet has also moved away from that traditional meat and two veg to having more access to convenience and takeaway foods'.

In 2016, the Department for Environment, Food & Rural Affairs (Defra) published historic data from its National Food Survey, highlighting the evolution of our national diet since

the 40s. It shows our transition from fresh, seasonal, locally produced ingredients, and how our appetite for quick and easy meals has increased since the mid-50s, when rationing ended. This evolution in what goes onto our plates was driven by factors like increasing access to fridges (so produce didn't need to be bought so regularly or locally and could be transported further), freezers and microwaves in the home, and more women going to work so having less time.

Our need for convenience in modern Britain has led to a growing reliance on mass produced, so-called ultra-processed foods. These now account for more than half of the UK's family food purchases, according to research by Cambridge University. But as well as offering a time-saving option, research suggests ultra-processed foods are associated with an increase in body mass index (BMI). However, large-scale population weight gain can't simply be blamed on sausage rolls and microwave meals – there is a risk of oversimplifying what is a hugely complex issue.

Paul Gately, professor of exercise and obesity at Leeds Beckett University, says: 'This term "ultra-processed" gets a lot of attention but, as a professor, I don't really know what that means, so I'm pretty sure most people out there don't either.' When we attempt to categorise food like this – as inherently good or bad – he adds, people just end up even more confused.

In reality, socioeconomic factors play a huge role in our rising collective weight – and population averages don't tell the whole story. 'When you look at it on a continuum of rich to poor, we're actually seeing reduced rates of obesity in more affluent communities, and very accelerated growth in more deprived communities. There's a big widening of the gap,' Professor Gately explains. This is because vulnerable and poorer communities have borne the brunt of austerity measures and the cost of living crisis for the last decade or so, he explains. The latest UK inflation figures, released on 16 November, show prices have risen 11 per cent in the year to October and food basics – low-fat milk, pasta, butter – have been hit particularly hard by the hike.

Food insecurity is associated with both obesity and malnutrition. While these two states may seem paradoxical, Ms Piggott says what we have in the UK is not in fact an 'obesity crisis' but a 'nutrition crisis' instead. With people's overall health affected by a lack of good quality nutrition available to them. 'We've got large disparities in terms of social demographics, and those who face more food insecurity are less able to have a healthy, balanced diet,' Ms Piggott explains. Research shows, for example, that food-insecure adults consume less fruit, vegetables and dairy products, and have lower intakes of vitamins A and B6, calcium, magnesium and zinc.

And convenience foods are not all created equal. Some do have high nutritional value, Ms Piggott says, but these tend not to be the most affordable or accessible options. Meanwhile the cheaper and more widely consumed versions are typically higher in fat, sugar and salt, and much lower in fibre, she says. Food insecurity is decreasing access to nutritional options.

'It's easy for politicians to come out saying a bag of potatoes is cheaper than a bag of chips, but you also need knowledge of how to cook those potatoes, access to cooking facilities, as well as the time and energy [to cook],' Ms Piggot explains. 'We often assume everybody's got a bank card or a car to do a big supermarket shop, or the finances, cooking and storage facilities to buy and prepare food in bulk – but not everybody does,' she says.

Despite these reasons for increasing cases of obesity, some argue that the notion the UK is getting fatter and fatter has been overstated. GP Dr Asher Larmie – who posts on social media as The Fat Doctor – says the idea has been grossly exaggerated. 'Since the year 2000, if you look at the trajectory of population weight, it has slowed right down,' they say. 'The world is getting fatter, every country gains a little bit of weight over time, but on average we're not massively gaining weight as people suggest we are,' Dr Larmie says. That said, they add, 'what we are seeing is bigger gains on the more extreme ends of the curve.'

Indeed, the statistics show that while rates of obesity increased steeply in Britain between 1993 and 2000, that increase has slowed since then. Professor Gately puts this down to the fact there was, 'a lot of talk in the 1990s but very little action, and then a lot of action and investment in solutions between around 2000 and 2008, before the [economic] crash.'

Looking globally, the UK has lower rates of obesity than countries like the USA, Mexico and Turkey, but does rank fourth among European countries. This may in part be down to cultural differences in food and activity habits compared with our continental neighbours, Professor Gately suggests. 'In the UK, generally we have a view of food as fuel, whereas in parts of Europe they attach more of a social dimension to mealtimes, so there's a level of investment in diet and sitting down as a family to eat together,' he says.

'In places like Amsterdam and Scandinavia we've also seen an investment in activity, like embedding cycling into the culture.' With children's meals, Ms Piggott points out that Brits also tend to opt for processed, oven-cooked options, while other countries and cultures give children a smaller version of what the adults are eating. That said, the rest of Europe is not immune to the same weight pressures as the UK. The World Health Organisation (WHO)'s 2022 Regional Obesity Report shows population weight is rising across Europe as well – for similar reasons to those seen in the UK.

Dr Larmie's view is that much of this is simply part of human evolution when faced with modern lifestyles. A report by the Government conducted in 2007 reached similar conclusions: 'People in the UK today don't have less willpower and are not more gluttonous than previous generations. Nor is their biology significantly different,' it states. 'Society, however, has radically altered over the past five decades. The pace of the technological revolution is outstripping human evolution and, for an increasing number of people, weight gain is the inevitable – and largely involuntary – consequence of exposure to a modern lifestyle,' it continues.

So is this really the new normal? Where do we go from here? For Professor Gately, progress towards decreasing obesity levels is hampered by the adversarial nature of the debate in the UK, and the way discussions about food, diet and obesity are often polarised in the media. 'Elsewhere in Europe there are some good, collaborative approaches between communities, governments, supermarkets, health groups and manufacturers. We just haven't got the environment to do that in the UK – there are too many voices going in different directions.' What will really help, he adds, is if we listen, understand where people are coming from and the challenges they face, and then act accordingly.

Meanwhile, Ms Piggott and Dr Larmie agree that shame, stigma, and our national obsession with dieting aren't helping. 'One of the biggest predictors for weight gain is dieting,' Ms Piggott says. Several studies from universities in the USA, including Harvard Medical School, show that most people who lose weight by dieting go on to regain the weight and then some, ending up heavier in the long-term than they started. 'If intentional weight loss causes people to gain weight, the fact people are dieting at an earlier and earlier age, and are dieting much more frequently than they used to, is having a profound effect,' Dr Larmie says.

What we need instead, they add, is a 'health at every size' approach, focused on balance and moderation, rather than the ultimate goal always being weight loss. 'I say to people do what you individually can manage, what's within your means,' says Dr Larmie. 'Fuel your body to function, and do exercise that's fun and feels good and has nothing to do with weight loss.'

17 November 2022

Renaming obesity won't fix weight stigma overnight. Here's what we really need to do

An article from The Conversation.

By Ravisha Jayawickrama, PhD candidate, School of Population Health, Curtin University, Blake Lawrence, Lecturer, Curtin School of Population Health, Curtin University & Briony Hill, Deputy Head, Health and Social Care Unit and Senior Research Fellow, Monash University

The stigma that surrounds people living in larger bodies is pervasive and deeply affects the people it's directed at. It's been described as one of the last acceptable forms of discrimination.

Some researchers think the term 'obesity' itself is part of the problem, and are calling for a name change to reduce stigma. They're proposing 'adipose-based chronic disease' instead.

We study the stigma that surrounds obesity – around the time of pregnancy, among health professionals and health students, and in public health more widely. Here's what's really needed to reduce weight stigma.

Weight stigma is common

Up to 42% of adults living in larger bodies experience weight stigma. This is when others have negative beliefs, attitudes, assumptions and judgements towards them, unfairly viewing them as lazy, and lacking in willpower or self-discipline.

People in larger bodies experience discrimination in many areas, including in the workplace, intimate and family relationships, education, health care and the media.

Weight stigma is associated with harms including increased cortisol levels (the main stress hormone in the body), negative body image, increased weight gain, and poor mental health. It leads to decreased uptake of, and quality of, health care.

Weight stigma may even pose a greater threat to someone's health than increasing body size.

Should we rename obesity?

Calls to remove or rename health conditions or identifications to reduce stigma are not new. For example, in the 1950s homosexuality was classed as a 'sociopathic personality disturbance'. Following many years of protests and activism, the term and condition were removed from the globally recognised classification of mental health disorders.

In recent weeks, European researchers have renamed non-alcoholic fatty liver disease 'metabolic dysfunction-associated steatotic liver disease'. This occurred after up to 66% of health-care professionals surveyed felt the terms 'non-alcoholic' and 'fatty' to be stigmatising.

Perhaps it is finally time to follow suit and rename obesity. But is 'adiposity-based chronic disease' the answer?

A new name needs to go beyond BMI

There are two common ways people view obesity.

First, most people use the term for people with a body-mass index (BMI) of 30kg/m² or above. Most, if not all, public health organisations also use BMI to categorise obesity and make assumptions about health.

However, BMI alone is not enough to accurately summarise someone's health. It does not account for muscle mass and does not provide information about the distribution of body weight or adipose tissue (body fat). A high BMI can occur without biological indicators of poor health.

Second, obesity is sometimes used to describe the condition of excess weight when mainly accompanied by metabolic abnormalities.

To simplify, this reflects how the body has adapted to the environment in a way that makes it more susceptible to health risks, with excess weight a by-product of this.

Renaming obesity 'adiposity-based chronic disease' acknowledges the chronic metabolic dysfunction associated with what we currently term obesity. It also avoids labelling people purely on body size.

Is obesity a disease anyway?

'Adiposity-based chronic disease' is an acknowledgement of a disease state. Yet there is still no universal consensus on whether obesity is a disease. Nor is there clear agreement on the definition of 'disease'.

People who take a biological-dysfunction approach to disease argue dysfunction occurs when physiological or psychological systems don't do what they're supposed to.

By this definition, obesity may not be classified as a disease until after harm from the additional weight occurs. That's because the excess weight itself may not initially be harmful.

Even if we do categorise obesity as a disease, there may still be value in renaming it.

Renaming obesity may improve public understanding that while obesity is often associated with an increase in BMI, the increased BMI itself is not the disease. This change could move the focus from obesity and body size, to a more nuanced understanding and discussion of the biological, environmental, and lifestyle factors associated with it.

Workshopping alternatives

Before deciding to rename obesity, we need discussions between obesity and stigma experts, health-care professionals, members of the public, and crucially, people living with obesity.

Such discussions can ensure robust evidence informs any future decisions, and proposed new terms are not also stigmatising.

What else can we do?

Even then, renaming obesity may not be enough to reduce the stigma.

Our constant exposure to the socially-defined and acceptable idealisation of smaller bodies (the 'thin ideal') and the pervasiveness of weight stigma means this stigma is deeply ingrained at a societal level.

Perhaps true reductions in obesity stigma may only come from a societal shift – away from the focus of the 'thin ideal' to one that acknowledges health and wellbeing can occur at a range of body sizes.

30 July 2023

THE CONVERSATION

Don't call people obese – it makes it harder for them to lose weight, researchers say

Labelling obesity 'chronic appetite dysregulation' might reduce some of the stigma attached to being overweight.

By Laura Donnelly, health editor

Obesity should be rebranded - to encourage people struggling with their weight, researchers say.

Scientists said those who struggled to resist temptation to overeat should be treated as though they have an illness - which they named 'chronic appetite dysregulation'. Such a move might reduce the stigma associated with obesity, they suggested, and help people to seek professional help with weight loss.

Scientists have identified hundreds of genes that increase the risk of obesity, and affect parts of the brain that control impulses and regulate appetite.

Researchers said people in this situation should be treated as suffering from a disease, which might make them more likely to access treatments.

Margaret Steele, a lecturer at the School of Public Health, University College Cork, said instead of focussing on body mass index, doctors should consider the physiological health of those with weight problems and how well they could function metabolically.

Working alongside the University of Galway, she studied the philosophical considerations about how obesity should be classified.

They concluded that excess weight alone was not in itself a disease - but said those with physiological health problems related to weight and who struggled to control excess eating should be treated as suffering from the illness 'chronic appetite dysregulation'.

Presenting her findings at the European Congress on Obesity in Dublin, Dr Steele said: 'If the public is confused about obesity, people living with obesity are more likely to face stigma and less likely to receive appropriate treatment.'

She said those with chronic appetite dysregulation found it harder to resist the temptation from an environment that 'throws so much food at us'.

'It's not a question of willpower, it's not a question of making decisions. It's at a much, much deeper level that we don't really have full control over. They're constantly getting signals that they're hungry and they feel physical hunger all the time. They're constantly being sent signals to eat and so they might respond by overeating.'

'These are the people that need to get some kind of medical help to not do that and these are the people with the disease.'

Not all fat people have 'the disease'

She added: 'Not everyone who's fat has the disease – it might just be that your setpoint weight is higher but there's nothing pathological going on. Equally, you can be thin and have the disease as well.'

The debate over whether obesity should be classed as a disease has gone on for decades, with the World Health Organisation classing it as such since 1936 while the NHS still refers to it as a term used to 'describe a person who has excess body fat'.

Critics say medicalising obesity by framing it as a disease rather than a consequence of behaviour, can be counterproductive, making people helpless about changing their lifestyles.

Dr Max Pemberton, a psychiatrist, said it 'takes away personal responsibility and places it with doctors'.

Comparing it to alcoholism and smoking, he said it is part of a wider trend to medicalise aspects of our life —turning individual decisions into a disease.

He said: 'People who are overweight and want to lose weight should be met with compassion and support. But we can be kind and caring to people who are struggling without claiming they have a disease. Disease suggests there is an inevitability when it does not have to be that way.

'There are generic components, just like there are genes that predispose people to be much more likely to become addicted to smoking than other people. But we would not classify smoking as a disease – it causes disease but we understand it as a behaviour that we have a choice in.

Genetic predisposition

'Even those who have a genetic predisposition to become fat are not slaves to their DNA. If we pathologize obesity, we fail to look at the complicated social factors that are involved and we almost stop considering the legislation and policy changes that are and can be made to address obesity.'

Prof Jason Halford, president of the European Association for the Study of Obesity, said many people with weight problems 'feel food is controlling them'.

He said the view that biology causes overconsumption of food 'remains controversial and is at odds with the view that obesity is a matter of individual responsibility' but was increasingly borne out by the evidence.

Dr Steele said: 'What people with obesity want and deserve is not necessarily a single neat disease diagnosis, but appropriate treatment, delivered respectfully, in a timely, affordable, and supportive way.

'Fatphobia runs very deep in our culture, and it's inextricably linked with classism, sexism, racism and other structures of oppression.'

18 May 2023

Why food deprivation in childhood is linked to obesity

An article from The Conversation.

By Khizra Tariq, PhD Candidate in the Nutrition, Psychopharmacology & Brain Development Unit, University of Salford

As energy prices rise and the cost of living goes up, it is estimated that there are 4 million children from poorer households who have limited or uncertain access to healthy food.

My current PhD research is examining how this childhood food insecurity affects eating behaviour. Research suggests that food deprivation in childhood leads to obesity.

A 2017 study found that children between the age of eight and ten from homes that do not have easy access to healthy food are five times more likely to be obese compared to those from households that have enough food.

The study, which looked at 50 mothers and their children, found that children in households where food scarcity is a problem ate food when they were not hungry and were more likely to eat five or more snacks per day.

This is what is known as the 'insurance hypothesis' – the theory is that people who do not have ready access to food eat more to store energy when they do have food, to avoid hunger in the future when food is scarce.

But another recent study conducted with 394 adults in the UK found no difference in the total energy intake of food-insecure and food-secure people. What it did find, though, was that the diet of people without ready access to healthy food was high in carbohydrates, with less fibre and protein than other people in the study.

The time gaps between when food-insecure people ate were also inconsistent when compared to those with ready access to healthy food. This could be due to financial reasons. The people who lacked access to food could not keep regular intervals between meals, but instead ate as food became available.

These research findings are concerning because eating high-calorie foods (often high in sugar and fats and classed as unhealthy food items) and skipping meals have been found to be linked with obesity.

It suggests that eating practices which result from food insecurity are factors that can lead to obesity.

The role of stress

The emotional toll of a childhood living in poverty may also lead to obesity. A 2018 research review of the factors leading to childhood obesity looked at the role played by family environment.

It suggests that low income, the inability to access or afford nutritious food and the stress caused by lack of income and food create a negative psychological and emotional environment for children. This family disharmony disrupts homeostasis – the body's ability to monitor and maintain its internal state.

Over time, this research suggests, this can lead to obesity. One way this can happen is through overeating to cope with stress – what is known as 'emotional eating' – when we use food to soothe or make ourselves feel better.

Increased stress levels cause dysregulation of certain peptides and hormones in the body, such as insulin, cortisol and ghrelin. In turn, higher levels of these hormones and peptides are associated with increased appetite for high-calorie foods.

Children are particularly affected because they are in the process of developing habits that will last into adulthood. Negative emotions cause changes in parts of the brain that are responsible for the development of habits and memory. If children eat comfort foods to reduce distress and this becomes a habit, they will use the same strategy to respond to future stress. Over time, this could lead to obesity.

Emotional eating

Other research studies have explored the link between emotional eating and obesity. A study conducted in 2019 with 150 adults explored the relationship between obesity and socioeconomic disadvantage, psychological distress and emotional eating.

It found that lower socioeconomic status was associated with higher distress, and that higher distress was associated with higher levels of emotional eating. In turn, higher emotional eating was associated with higher BMI.

Research carried out at the University of Salford with more than 600 adults also found that that food insecurity was associated with a poorer diet, and that greater distress and eating to cope was linked with higher BMI.

This research was conducted with adults rather than looking at the childhood causes of obesity. But it suggests that psychological distress and subsequent emotional eating is a pathway that links poverty with obesity.

What's more, a study carried out in the US with 676 adolescents from diverse backgrounds found that perceived stress, worries and confused mood were associated with emotional eating.

In the UK, 29% of men and 27% of women are obese. This rate will be higher in the coming years if more is not done to protect children living in poverty.

11 January 2023

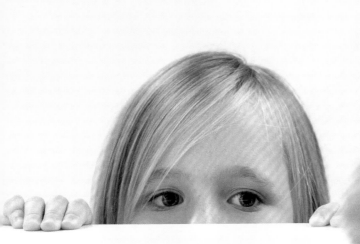

Is the UK Government's childhood obesity programme working?

How has the UK Government's National Child Measurement Programme (NCMP), designed to tackle childhood obesity, impacted child and parent mental health?

The Queen Mary University of London has researched England's National Measurement Programme (NCMP), an intervention designed to tackle childhood obesity, to better understand the experiences of parents and their children categorised as 'overweight' and 'very overweight'.

The results conclude that the current programme may actually harm the children it aims to help.

What is the UK Government's National Child Measurement Programme (NCMP)?

The UK Government's National Child Measurement Programme (NCMP) records the height and weight of school children in England. Its purpose is to gather relevant data so the Government can understand long-term trends in childhood obesity. This information is used to inform national and local initiatives.

Through the programme, primary school-aged children are weighed and measured at school by visiting health professionals. Their Body Mass Index (BMI) is calculated, and the results are issued to parents to advise whether their child has been categorised as:

- 'Underweight'
- 'Healthy weight'
- 'Overweight'
- 'Very overweight'

The Queen Mary study is the first to focus on childhood obesity as experienced by children and parents

The Queen Mary study is the first to focus on the experiences of children and parents who were categorised as 'overweight' or 'very overweight'.

The study analysis pointed to a significant degree of concern exhibited by these families regarding the potential mental health impact on their children.

Perhaps most prominently, the label of 'overweight' or 'very overweight' triggered the child's overnight awareness of body weight. This permanently altered their relationship with food and their relation to their peers.

What is the mental health impact on overweight and obese children?

Taking part in the programme designed to reduce childhood obesity was an emotionally significant moment for many children who were told they were above a healthy weight.

Those children reported feeling anxious and embarrassed about getting weighed, the result, and the potential for teasing. Some parents dismissed the result.

Are potential mental health disorders and unhealthy dieting behaviours more dangerous than the weight itself?

Many parents expressed concern that the potential for mental health disorders, eating disorders and unhealthy dieting behaviours in the future was 'far more dangerous than the weight itself', and their priority was the child's happiness.

These concerns are not unfounded – the study cites an analysis of the impact of weight-related conversations on children, which found that being encouraged to lose weight, teasing, and weight-related criticism was associated with poorer self-perceptions, increased dieting and dysfunctional eating behaviours.

Further research is needed to understand whether parents' concerns are being borne out in the long term and to find ways to mitigate any negative effects of the programme. In

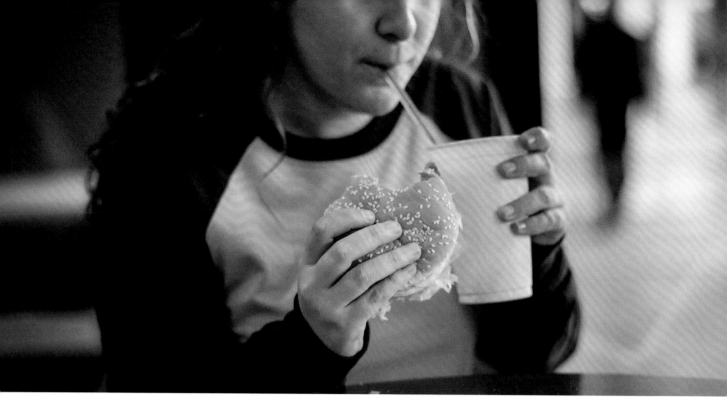

some areas of England, efforts have been made to change the wording of the results letters issued to families, for example, to avoid using stigmatising words like 'overweight' and 'obese'. But these measures are locally driven and vary across the country.

Is the National Child Measurement Programme in its current form causing some children harm, how can this be mitigated, and how does it balance against the positive use of the data the programme produces?

The Queen Mary authors say policymakers need to thoroughly consider the questions that their findings raise: is the National Child Measurement Programme in its current form causing some children harm, how can this be mitigated, and how does it balance against the positive use of the data the programme produces?

The NCMP generates valuable insights, but it requires policy and actions – beyond those which can be taken by families acting alone – to halt and reverse the rising proportion of children who are an unhealthy weight.

Childhood obesity strongly linked to child poverty

What is extremely important to remember is that childhood obesity is strongly linked to child poverty. It begs the question, do initiatives like this actually help children? Or does it further stigma and promote unhealthy body image and eating disorders?

According to this study, there is little evidence that initiatives to change the behaviour of individual families are successful in reducing childhood obesity at a population level.

Policy approaches to tackling obesity, including the soft drinks industry levy, and extending eligibility for free school meals as recommended in the National Food Strategy independent review, may be much more ethical and effective.

The food industry and poverty must be addressed

Dr Meredith K.D. Hawking, lead author and Research Fellow at Queen Mary University of London, commented:

'Many parents have legitimate concerns about the impact the National Child Measurement Programme might have on children's self-perception and food practices as they grow older. More research is needed to understand whether these concerns are borne out in the long term and to find ways to mitigate them if the programme is to continue.

'Without meaningful regulation of the food industry or measures to address poverty, parents will be unsupported in their efforts to help children live healthier lives'

'To improve child health, the Government must act on the evidence the NCMP and other sources are producing. We know that childhood obesity is a strong indicator of child poverty. Without meaningful regulation of the food industry or measures to address poverty, parents will be unsupported in their efforts to help children live healthier lives.'

10 February 2023

Consider...

Do you think that the National Child Measurement Programme could be damaging to a child's mental health?

How do you think it can affect a child? Write down some of your ideas.

www.openaccessgovernment.org

The economics of obesity

Reducing obesity is not just good for our health, it's good for the economy too.

By Lydia Leon

Rates of obesity have nearly doubled in recent decades. In 2019 over 28% of UK adults and a quarter of children in year 6 were obese. Food-related ill health, including high BMI, is second only to smoking as a contributor to poor health outcomes in the UK.

This is strongly shaped by the food-environment. Inequalities in food-related illnesses are stark and widening: in the most deprived areas in England, prevalence of obesity is around 17 percentage points higher than in the least deprived.

Why does this matter?

Obesity increases the risk of many preventable diseases including type 2 diabetes, cardiovascular disease and some cancers. Additionally, obesity can reduce life expectancy, sometimes by up to nine years – an effect comparable to that of smoking.

But obesity is not just a health issue. A recent study by Frontier Economics has strengthened the case for tackling obesity by quantifying the huge economic costs associated with its impacts on individual quality of life, as well as the pressure it puts on health care services and the wider economy.

The report estimated that the annual cost of adult obesity to UK society is around £54 billion, roughly equivalent to 2-3% of GDP or the total annual funding allocated to schools in England.

Three quarters of the Frontier Economics estimate comes from putting a monetary value on the number of healthy life years lost (either to premature death or ill health) due to obesity using measures known as QALYs (quality adjusted life years). This value is incredibly important to society, even if it's not directly cashable savings.

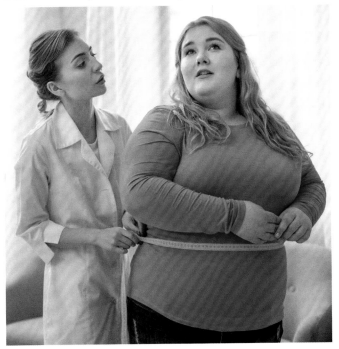

The costs of obesity are not just experienced by individuals. According to the Frontier Economics report, the NHS spends around £6.5 billion a year (close to 4% of its 22/23 budget) on treating its consequences. The King's Fund forecasts that this will increase to £10 billion a year by 2050.

> 'The NHS spends around £6.5 billion a year on treating the consequences of obesity.'

High rates of obesity also result in significant indirect costs to the economy beyond the health sector. Reductions in workforce productivity and increased use of social care are estimated to cost around £7.5 billion a year.

What needs to be done?

The most cost-effective approach to tackling obesity-related ill health is to prevent its rise to begin with.

The first official recognition of obesity as a serious issue requiring a public health response was three decades ago in the 1991 *Health of the Nation* report. In the years since, despite over a dozen government strategies, hundreds of wide-ranging policy proposals and growing public concern, rates of obesity have only increased.

Too many policies have relied on individual will power or voluntary action from industry to turn the tide. In an environment in which the healthy option is rarely the easy option, it is unsurprising that these approaches have had minimal impact.

We need low-agency obesity-prevention policies that take a population-wide approach and ensure affordable and nutritious food is easily accessible for everyone.

A recent report by the Behavioural Insights Team and Impact on Urban Health examined the economic cost benefit of four such policies that were either recently implemented by the UK government or scheduled for future implementation. The policies included restricting the locations of foods high in fat, salt, and sugar (HFSS) in stores and the Soft Drinks Industry Levy, as well as planned restrictions on HFSS multibuy options and advertising.

> 'The benefits of four obesity-prevention policies could provide a combined net return to the UK economy of £76 billion over 25 years.'

The report used Government impact assessments of expected costs (eg, enforcement costs for the taxpayer or transition costs for industry) and benefits of the four policy options to estimate a combined net return to the UK economy of £76 billion over 25 years. The benefits included individual improvements in quality of life, savings to the NHS and social care, as well as projected gains in workforce productivity due to a healthier population. Since estimates outlined in the report only included data available in the

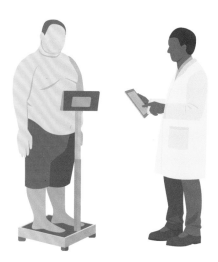

Government's own impact assessments, which did not always capture the full range of likely benefits, the net return estimate is likely to be a very conservative estimate. To give a sense of scale, an independent academic estimate for the sugar tax put the daily calorie reduction at 17.8kcal per person, which the UK government's own tool would estimate at a value of £9.5 billion over 25 years.

As well as providing significant returns for the public purse, approaches that take the focus away from unhealthy food need not be detrimental to business and their bottom lines. This is no clearer than in the success of the 2018 Soft Drinks Industry Levy (SDIL) which has improved public health and protected industry profits. Whilst the total sugar purchased per household from drinks subject to the SDIL has declined by around a third (and was greatest in groups with lowest income), the total sales of drinks subject to the levy increased by a fifth since its implementation. These gains, many of which have been possible due to significant reformulation of products by industry, are in stark contrast to reported progress towards the Government's voluntary sugar reduction targets in which only a 3.5% average reduction in sugar has been observed.

In 2020, the National Food Strategy called for a new salt and sugar tax to replace the SDIL which it suggests could reduce average calorie consumption by 15-38 kcal a day and save tens of thousands of lives, whilst bringing in around £3 billion in tax revenue. Despite frequent claims to the contrary, public support for these kinds of obesity interventions is high. One recent poll found that 63% of people in the UK would support the expansion of the sugar tax from soft drinks to foods such as sweets and biscuits. What are we waiting for?

8 December 2022

Brainstorm

Around £6.5 billion a year is spent by the NHS on treating the consequences of obesity.

In small groups, brainstorm some ways that the NHS could reduce this amount. How do you think they could improve the health of the population?

Sugary drinks tax may have prevented over 5,000 cases of obesity a year in year six girls alone

The introduction of the soft drinks industry levy – the 'sugary drinks tax' – in England was followed by a drop in the number of cases of obesity among older primary school children, according to Cambridge researchers. Taking into account current trends in obesity, their estimates suggest that around 5,000 cases of obesity per year may have been prevented in year six girls alone.

The study, published today in PLOS Medicine, looked at the impact of the levy on reception age children and those in year six, but found no significant association between the levy and obesity levels in year six boys or younger children from reception class.

The research was supported by the National Institute of Health and Care Research (NIHR) and the Medical Research Council.

Obesity has become a global public health problem. In England, one in ten reception age children (four to five years old) is living with obesity and this figure doubles

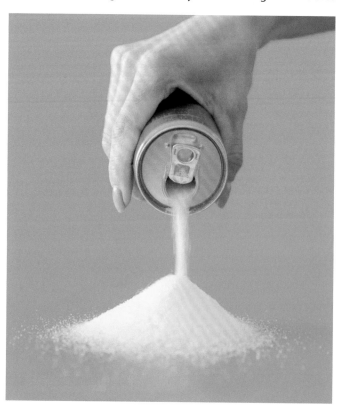

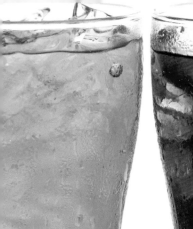
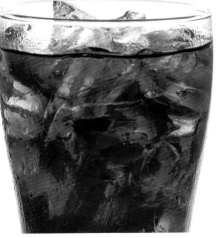
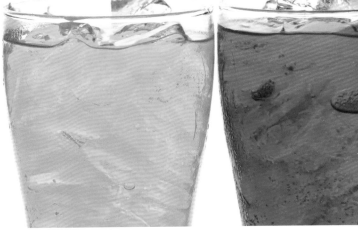

to one in five children in year six (10 to 11 years). Children who are obese are more likely to suffer from serious health problems including high blood pressure, type II diabetes and depression in childhood and in later life.

In the UK, young people consume significantly more added sugars than is recommended – by late adolescence, they typically consume 70g of added sugar per day, more than double the recommended amount (30g). A large source of this is sugar-sweetened drinks. Children from deprived households are more likely to be at risk of obesity and to be heavy consumers of sugar-sweetened drinks.

In April 2018, to protect children from excessive sugar consumption and tackle childhood obesity, the UK governments introduced a two-tier sugar tax on soft drinks – the soft drinks industry levy. The tax was targeted at manufacturers of the drinks to incentivise them to reduce the sugar content of soft drinks.

Researchers from the Medical Research Council (MRC) Epidemiology Unit at the University of Cambridge tracked changes in the levels of obesity in children in England in reception year and year six between 2014 and 2020. Taking account of previous trends in obesity levels, they compared changes in levels of obesity 19 months after the sugar tax came into effect.

The team found that the introduction of the sugar tax was associated with an 8% relative reduction* in obesity levels in year six girls, equivalent to preventing 5,234 cases of obesity per year in this group alone. Reductions were greatest in girls whose schools were in deprived areas, where children are known to consume the largest amount of sugary drinks – those living in the most deprived areas saw a 9% reduction.

However, the team found no associations between the sugar tax coming into effect and changes in obesity levels in children from reception class. In year 6 boys, there was no overall change in obesity prevalence.

Dr Nina Rogers from the MRC Epidemiology Unit at Cambridge, the study's first author, said: 'We urgently need to find ways to tackle the increasing numbers of children living with obesity, otherwise we risk our children growing up to face significant health problems. That was one reason why the UK's soft drinks industry levy was introduced, and the evidence so far is promising. We've shown for the first time that it is likely to have helped prevent thousands of children each year becoming obese.

'It isn't a straightforward picture, though, as it was mainly older girls who benefited. But the fact that we saw the biggest difference among girls from areas of high deprivation is important and is a step towards reducing the health inequalities they face.'

Although the researchers found an association rather than a causal link, this study adds to previous findings that the levy was associated with a substantial reduction in the amount of sugar in soft drinks.

Senior author Professor Jean Adams from the MRC Epidemiology Unit said: 'We know that consuming too many sugary drinks contributes to obesity and that the UK soft drinks levy led to a drop in the amount of sugar in soft drinks available in the UK, so it makes sense that we also see a drop in cases of obesity, although we only found this in girls. Children from more deprived backgrounds tend to consume the largest amount of sugary drinks, and it was among girls in this group that we saw the biggest change.'

There are several reasons why the sugar tax did not lead to changes in levels of obesity among the younger children, they say. Very young children consume fewer sugar-sweetened drinks than older children, so the soft drinks levy would have had a smaller effect. Similarly, fruit juices are not included in the levy, but contribute similar amounts of sugar in young children's diets as sugar-sweetened beverages.

It's unclear why the sugar tax might affect obesity prevalence in girls and boys differently, however, especially since boys are higher consumers of sugar-sweetened beverages. One explanation the researchers put forward is the possible impact of advertising – numerous studies have found that boys are often exposed to more food advertising content than girls, both through higher levels of TV viewing and in how adverts are framed. Physical activity is often used to promote junk food and boys, compared to girls, have been shown to be more likely to believe that energy dense junk foods depicted in adverts will boost physical performance and so are more likely to choose energy-dense, nutrient-poor products following celebrity endorsements.

The study was a collaboration involving researchers from the University of Cambridge, London School of Hygiene and Tropical Medicine, University of Oxford, Great Ormond Street Institute of Child Health and University of Bath.

*A relative reduction is the difference between the expected incidence of obesity had the sugar tax not been introduced and the actual incidence.

26 January 2023

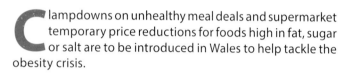

Wales to clamp down on junk food meal deals to tackle obesity

Welsh government says it will go further than UK government's plans for England in trying to encourage healthier eating.

By Steven Morris

Clampdowns on unhealthy meal deals and supermarket temporary price reductions for foods high in fat, sugar or salt are to be introduced in Wales to help tackle the obesity crisis.

With almost two-thirds of adults in Wales overweight or obese, the Labour-led government announced it would go further than England in framing laws designed to tackle the promotion of ultra-processed foods.

The government said it intended to match the UK government's plans to curb volume promotions such as buy one get one free in England. It also revealed proposals to tackle meal deals and temporary price reductions, arguing it needed to do more because of the scale of the crisis.

The Welsh deputy minister for mental health and wellbeing, Lynne Neagle, said: 'Rising levels of obesity are creating the serious burden of preventable ill health in Wales. The situation is urgent and we have to act now.

'We're not banning meal deals but we want to shift the focus of meal deals towards healthier, more nutritionally balanced food. Lots of them come with large bags of crisps and the snacks are often high in fat and sugar. We want to make sure we can still have meal deals available at an affordable price but which are not so high in calories, fat and sugar.'

Research from Public Health Wales found that three-quarters of lunchtime meal deals exceed the recommended level of calories and salt for lunch.

The least healthy lunchtime options contain two-thirds of daily calorie intake, more than 122% of daily fat intake, 149% of sugar and 112% of salt. The majority of dinnertime meal combinations exceed average energy requirements.

The researchers concluded that if someone bought an average meal deal for lunch five days a week, they would gain more than 6lbs (2.8kg) in a year. If they bought a high-calorie meal deal for lunch five days a week, they could gain 47lbs (21kg) in a year.

Neagle said the government would not ban temporary price reductions either but added: 'Our aim is to rebalance our food environments so that the healthy choice becomes the easy choice.'

Last week, the UK government put off by two years its planned ban on buy one get one free junk food deals, citing the cost of living crisis. The Welsh government is planning to bring in its restrictions by 2025 and said it would press ahead even if the UK government did not.

Neagle said: 'It would be great if England went ahead with these plans. We think that alignment across the UK is helpful but we have a responsibility to do what we can to tackle the crisis that we're facing in Wales now.'

She denied this was an example of the nanny state. 'Tackling obesity is not just about personal responsibility. It's about the food environment in which we live, which is full of processed, unhealthy food.'

The regulations will apply to major outlets and the government will also look at curbing unhealthy food bought online and offers involving loyalty cards.

The Welsh government said 62% of people in Wales aged 16 and over were overweight or obese.

The Welsh Conservatives' James Evans, the shadow minister for mental health and wellbeing, said: 'We need cast iron assurances from the Welsh Labour government that they do not intend to ban meal deals and that any new regulations will not increase the average weekly cost for shoppers.'

27 June 2023

Curbing appetites for ultra-processed foods

Ultra-processed foods have been linked to a range of health implications, but the level of consumption remains high. We spoke to researchers at Imperial College London to find out why.

The causes of overweight and obesity are often multifaceted and driven by both genetic and environmental factors. At a basic level, obesity and overweight result from an energy imbalance in the amount of calories consumed and expended. According to the World Health Organization (WHO), the rate of obesity has tripled worldwide since 1975, alongside an increase in the prevalence and consumption of micronutrient-poor and ultra-processed foods. Rising food prices and political inertia to promote healthier food options mean many families are reaching for the cheapest – and often least healthy – products, posing considerable implications for their long-term health. Children in particular are consuming high amounts of ultra-processed foods, leaving them at greater risk of maintaining unhealthy eating patterns when they reach adulthood. To discuss this further, Lorna Rothery spoke to Dr Kiara Chang and Dr Eszter Vamos from Imperial College London's School of Public Health.

Can you outline the impact of obesity, and the secondary conditions associated with it, on the economy and health services in the UK?

Obesity is a global public health challenge and an important risk factor for type 2 diabetes, heart disease and some cancers. The UK has one of the highest rates of obesity, with one in three adults living with obesity and another third overweight. An estimated £6.1 million was spent on overweight and obesity by the UK's National Health Service in 2014-2015, and the wider economic costs to society are estimated at £27 billion.

How far can the consumption of unhealthy and ultra-processed foods be linked to increasing levels of obesity across the UK? How do you expect the cost-of-living crisis will affect this?

Evidence from a randomised controlled trial shows that ultra-processed food consumption causes weight gain and excess calorie intake. Our previous research using large-scale and UK-based longitudinal data found a link between higher consumption of ultra-processed foods and increased risk of obesity and type 2 diabetes in adults and more rapid weight gain and body fat gain in children.

These foods are often relatively cheap, and during the cost-of-living crisis, many families struggle to access healthy foods with long-lasting effects on health. We need to make healthier foods more available and accessible for low-income households through subsidies and price promotions while taking action to restrict the marketing of ultra-processed foods.

Your research on ultra-processed food content of school meals and packed lunches in the UK noted that British

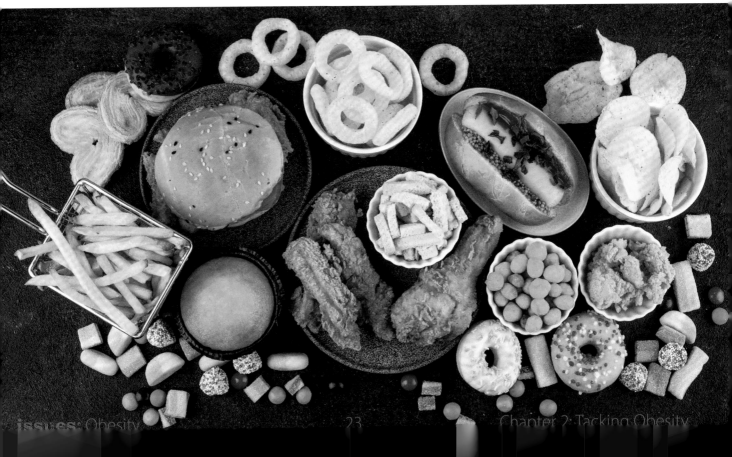

children have the highest levels of ultra-processed food consumption in Europe. What are some of the key factors driving this?

The UK is a leading consumer of ultra-processed foods in Europe. British children consume, on average, 65% of their daily calorie intake from these foods; this is much higher than British adults, who consume 54% of their daily calorie intake from ultra-processed foods. There may be multiple factors contributing to this high level of consumption. Ultra-processed foods are typically designed to be hyper-palatable but have a low satiety potential and are more prone to over-consumption (we can eat a lot of them without feeling full). They are widely available and very convenient as they are ready to be consumed. Ultra-processed foods are also aggressively marketed with strong brands and especially target children (e.g., using cartoon characters on the packaging or advertising free toys). They are relatively cheap due to the use of low-cost ingredients in their production, and they are often marketed as healthy options.

In some of the world's most developed economies, ultra-processed foods make up a significant proportion of people's diets; do you think there is enough public understanding of the negative health impacts associated with their consumption? If not, why?

Consumption levels are highest in high-income countries but are rising most rapidly in low- and middle-income countries. Although public awareness has increased about the negative effects associated with their consumption, it is not always easy for consumers to recognise ultra-processed foods. Currently, the front-of-pack food labelling does not indicate how foods are processed. A practical way to identify them is to check if the list of ingredients includes food additives or anything that we do not usually use in home cooking (e.g., high-fructose corn syrup, hydrogenated oils, flavour enhancers, thickeners, etc.). These are often substances we are unfamiliar with and cannot even recognise as consumers. If at least one of these substances is included in the ingredients, it indicates that the product is ultra-processed.

The UK Government was criticised for delaying plans to ban pre-watershed TV advertising for junk food; what should be done at the policy level to promote healthier eating?

Aggressive advertising is a primary driver of the consumption of unhealthy foods, and the UK government's decision to delay decisive actions to restrict junk food advertising is a missed opportunity. Since UK adults and children are leading consumers of ultra-processed foods globally, bold policy actions would be required to reduce their harmful health effects. For example, mandatory front-of-pack labelling on ultra-processed foods would assist consumers in selecting healthier food options. Fiscal policies that increase the price of ultra-processed foods and subsidise minimally processed foods and freshly prepared meals could promote the consumption of healthier and more nutritious foods. Updating public food procurement policies (government purchasing food or food services) could help prioritise locally sourced fresh foods and minimally processed foods while restricting the supply of ultra-processed foods.

Originally published in issue 25 of Health Europa Quarterly. By Dr Kiara Chang, Research Fellow and Dr Eszter Vamos, Clinical Senior Lecturer, Imperial College London www.imperial.ac.uk

20 March 2023

Design

Design a poster highlighting what ultra-processed foods are, and their negative effects.

Consider...

British children consume, on average, 65% of their daily calorie intake from ultra-processed foods.

Have a look at the foods you eat over three days. How much ultra-processed food have you eaten? Are you more likely to eat ultra-processed food at certain meal times? Is there any way you can reduce the amount you eat?

Research

Have a look at some of the foods you have at home. Look at the list of ingredients, are there any that you don't recognise?

See what information you can find out about the ingredients. What is their purpose in the food?

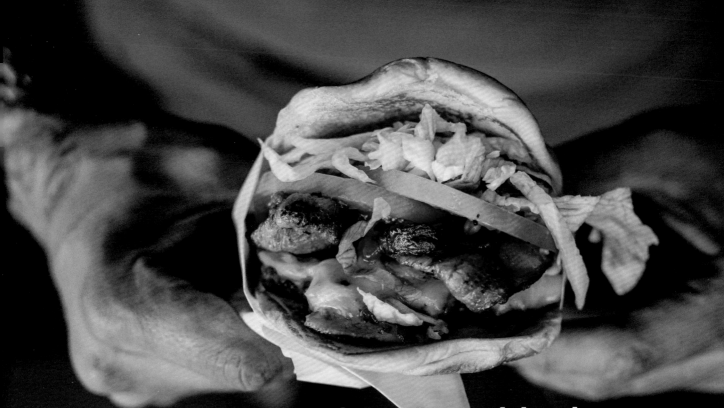

'I'm a doctor – here's how I would solve Britain's obesity crisis'

From a GP to the head of the behavioural 'nudge' unit, three professionals give their opinions on how to tackle our weight problem.

By Charlotte Lytton

For 30 years, curtailing obesity rates in Britain has made it onto successive prime ministers' agendas – yet it's proven to be the nettle none can grasp. Fourteen strategies, 689 policies and a further 14 bodies specifically set up (and then disbanded) later, waistlines in the UK are only growing, with nothing seemingly able to halt the trend.

A report this week found that menu calorie counts, introduced with the idea of encouraging customers to cut back, are often way off the actual number of calories contained, making it appear little more than a tick-box exercise. Boris Johnson's plan to ban junk food deals has also been scrapped, with Rishi Sunak saying that a cost of living crisis is no time to further increase food prices. At the same time, obesity now affects two thirds of UK adults, at a cost of £6billion to the NHS each year.

The current Government's manifesto pledged to give everyone 'five extra years of healthy, independent life by 2035 and to narrow the gap between the richest and the poorest', as well as promising to halve child obesity and reduce the condition among adults – yet current figures suggest we have never been further from the mark. Here's what three experts think we should do to ensure a healthier future …

The behaviourist

Prof David Halpern

President of the Behavioural Insights Team

'Let's give the power back to the consumer and ask them what they want'

We're the fat men and women of Europe, and we broadly know what kinds of choices we need to make to put that right. Yet instead we are leaving the NHS to pick up the pieces of our unhealthy lifestyles, and spending an absolute fortune on the likes of diabetes treatment, cutting off limbs and pulling out teeth. We need to be able to have a mature conversation about overriding the current situation – created by an evolution of our genes and behaviours, and market dynamics – in order to achieve lasting change.

I head up the Behavioural Insights Team, also known as the Nudge unit, which was set up by the Government in 2010 with the idea that nudging people towards better choices without regulation or force is the best way to spark change long term. (We are now fully owned by Nesta, a charity.) We suggested nudges, such as the sugar tax in 2014 (implemented in 2018), and placing high-calorie foods away from checkouts in supermarkets. We also backed junk food advertising bans and an end to buy-one-get-one-free deals on such products, which were both announced as Government mandates – and then withdrawn. This week I have also co-signed the Covenant for Health, a paper outlining the policies that can reform the nation's health over five to 10 years, including a sugar and salt reformulation tax, which could help to cut daily caloric intake and halve obesity prevalence by 2030.

People may not like the idea of nudging, but while they'll say they want to be healthier, our environment makes it hard to achieve that, so it's right to make these kinds of changes on a wider level. We should be comfortable making tweaks that are in line with people's long-term desires that will ensure the health and wealth of the country.

It is evident that information, exercise and willpower will not reduce levels of obesity. What we need is upstream interventions that address the underlying factors that lead to poor health. I believe that people want to live more healthily, but this requires making it as easy and thoughtless to pick the option that's good for you as it currently is to select the one that isn't. We know some of these nudges have worked: reformulating drinks following the introduction of the sugar tax has led to a rise in lower-sugar soft drinks sales (meaning business interests and, to a degree, health is protected), and we could do more. Many of us order food online now, and changing a regular-sized meal to mean 'small' could also lead to a reduction in calorie consumption. These might not seem like major changes, perhaps the equivalent to eating one less chocolate bar a day, but the cumulative impact would be vast.

I don't believe this is tantamount to a nanny state, but the reverse: let's give the power back to the consumer, and ask

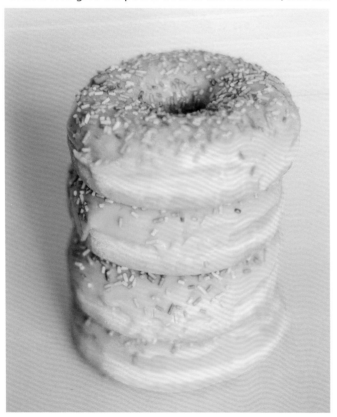

them what changes they think should be made, rather than getting hung up on personal responsibility or lambasting people for not paying attention or exercising enough. Asking people what they want, and giving individuals access to information procured by industry groups, the Government and researchers, will allow everyone to make up their own minds about how to shape our environment, and our future.

The GP

Prof Kamila Hawthorne

Chair of the Royal College of General Practitioners

'GPs need to show patients they're committed to helping them lose weight'

Two thirds of adults are overweight or obese in Britain, and as doctors, we're worried about what this means for the future of chronic diseases. We need to raise healthy food and healthy eating on the nation's list of priorities, and to do this together.

That starts with GP services, who need more resources to be able to support their patients in losing weight to improve their health. We need better access to dietitians and to psychological support to help people lose weight – it isn't an easy thing to do, and neither is keeping the weight off once it has been lost.

GPs can and already do play an important role in curbing obesity, by taking the time to show patients how committed we are as their doctors to helping them lose the weight that they need to lose, and convincing them that it's actually worth doing. I only get to spend 15 minutes with a patient – other GPs will likely have less time – and for the rest of the day, they're surrounded by all kinds of other influences. What I would really love is if they left my surgery and saw a public health campaign advertised on a bus, reiterating the benefits of weight loss, building on what we're doing in consultations.

I often say to people that if they can make these changes for themselves, they can do more for their health than any doctor can.

I work in a post-industrial town in the Welsh Valleys, and the high street is full of fast-food outlets. Obesity is closely linked to poverty, and ensuring healthy, low-carb and low-fat foods are accessible and local would make it far simpler for people to make better meals at home. There is a common perception that eating well is too expensive, particularly in a cost of living crisis, and that shouldn't be the case.

Teaching people how to eat well is vital, and we need to start this education young, because by the time I see patients with chronic conditions who are already very overweight, it's much harder to reverse the negative health outcomes that could have been avoided in the first place. In my view, prevention is far better than dealing with the aftermath.

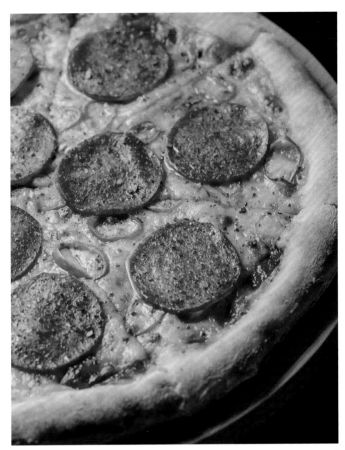

The anti-upf evangelist

Dr Chris van Tulleken

Author of 'Ultra Processed People'

'We need a revolution and to treat food companies like tobacco companies'

We are in the grip of a child health emergency – one that's been steadily growing for three decades – and I'm not sure we're doing anything much about it. We know that what drives weight gain and other diet-related diseases in this country is eating foods that are ultra-processed, high in fat, salt and sugar; yet at the moment, children see marketing for all of the above everywhere they turn. When they go into any shop, when they walk down any street, on their bus tickets, on their music apps, on their games that are funded by the food industry, their televisions, on YouTube. The situation that we've allowed to develop is absurd, unaffordable and morally repellent.

We need a revolution, and my proposal is simple: treat food companies like tobacco companies. They sell addictive products that they know damage human health, and they market them to vulnerable people; they also fund research, skewing it in their favour – which is no more valid than a tobacco company paying for studies. We need to make real food affordable and accessible for people, and to restrict the marketing of ultra-processed, high fat, salt and sugar foods. This is not anti-growth – the pharmaceutical industry, which is tightly regulated, has seen huge economic success since stricter guidelines were brought in, and the same can be done here.

Education around nutrition is important, but ultimately comes in relatively low on my list: there's less value in teaching children what they should be eating if they can't afford to do so in the first place, or are surrounded by aggressive marketing telling them to pick up the foods that are contributing to excess weight, which is the leading cause of death globally.

Countries like Mexico, Colombia and Brazil are beginning to better label food – they don't use our confusing traffic-light system, rather big black hexagons on unhealthy products, so you can spot them immediately. They also ban cartoon characters on packaging, to make them less appealing to children.

We need to avoid eating rubbish food from cradle to grave. At the moment, people don't have a choice.

Practical tips to trim the fat

Rewire your brain for weight loss

Do the jellied-eel test

'Before you eat, ask yourself, "Am I actually hungry?" Would you eat a jellied eel, or anything else you dislike, if that was to hand?' says nutritionist and weight-loss coach Pippa Hill. 'If the answer is no, drink a glass of water instead.' Lots of us eat when we're bored, but that feeling will pass, along with the urge to grab a biscuit.

Always eat proper meals – at a table

'If you graze in front of the television, you'll keep eating and finish the packet,' says Hill. 'In the 1970s we didn't eat like that. We had breakfast, lunch and dinner, that was it.'

You can't exercise away a bad diet

'Your body weight is 80 per cent diet, 15 per cent exercise and 5 per cent genetics,' says Hill. 'Exercise alone won't get your weight down.'

Think: 'Daytime need, nighttime greed'

During the day we need energy and at night we need to give our digestive system a rest and let it wind down for sleep. Don't eat after 8pm, 7pm if you can.

Can the diet drinks

'Sweeteners cause our bodies to release insulin. They make you crave sugar and don't help you lose weight,' says Hill. If you're thirsty drink water, or a cup of tea

22 July 2023

Artificial sweeteners do not help you lose weight, WHO warns

Consumption of free sugars is linked to rising obesity and increased cases of diabetes, cardiovascular diseases, cancer and tooth decay.

By Ella Pickover

People should avoid using sweeteners to help with weight control, global health leaders have said.

Low or no-calorie sweeteners are used instead of sugar to sweeten foods and drinks and can be found in products including desserts and ready meals, cakes, drinks, chewing gum and toothpaste.

Many people also add non-sugar sweeteners to their own food and beverages as a sugar alternative.

But new guidance from the World Health Organization (WHO) urges people not to use non-sugar sweeteners (NSS) as a tool for weight control.

It said consumption of free sugars has been linked to rising numbers of people who are overweight or obese as well as increases in cases of type two diabetes, cardiovascular diseases, cancer and tooth decay.

With a focus on reducing sugar intake, the WHO said 'interest in non-sugar sweeteners as a possible alternative has intensified'.

Because of the ability of artificial and natural sweeteners to impart a sweet taste without calories, some have argued they can help to prevent people becoming overweight or obese.

'This report highlights that universal replacement of sugar with sweeteners is not necessarily ideal, as this alone is unlikely to improve diet quality and produce the necessary changes to control weight long term' – Dr Duane Mellor, Aston Medical School

But others have suggested they may increase risk.

As a result, the WHO undertook a review of studies that have examined the impacts of sweeteners.

In all, WHO researchers examined data from 283 studies conducted in adults, children, pregnant women or mixed populations.

It said the results suggest the 'use of NSS does not confer any long-term benefit in reducing body fat in adults or children'.

But the authors said that in the short term, NSS use may lead to minor weightloss 'when their use leads to a reduction in total energy intake'.

The WHO also said there could be 'undesirable effects' linked to long-term use, such as an increased risk of type two diabetes, cardiovascular diseases and death.

But the authors said further research is needed.

'Replacing free sugars with NSS does not help with weight control in the long term,' said Francesco Branca, the WHO's director for nutrition and food safety.

'People need to consider other ways to reduce free sugars intake, such as consuming food with naturally occurring sugars, like fruit, or unsweetened food and beverages.

'NSS are not essential dietary factors and have no nutritional value.

'People should reduce the sweetness of the diet altogether, starting early in life, to improve their health.'

As a result of the study, the WHO released a new conditional guideline recommending against the use of NSS to control body weight or reduce the risk of noncommunicable diseases.

The recommendation applies to everyone except those with pre-existing diabetes.

It also applies to personal care and hygiene products containing NSS, such as toothpaste, skin cream, and medications.

Commenting on the guideline, Dr Duane Mellor, registered dietitian and senior lecturer at Aston Medical School, said: 'Overall this report highlights that universal replacement of sugar with sweeteners is not necessarily ideal, as this alone is unlikely to improve diet quality and produce the necessary changes to control weight long term.

'It is probably best not to stick with sugars to avoid sweeteners though – the answer is to try and reduce sugar intake.

'For some, that might include using small amounts of sweeteners in foods and drinks as a way to reduce overall sugar intake.

'Sweeteners may still have a place as a transitional or stepping stone to help people reduce their sugar intake.'

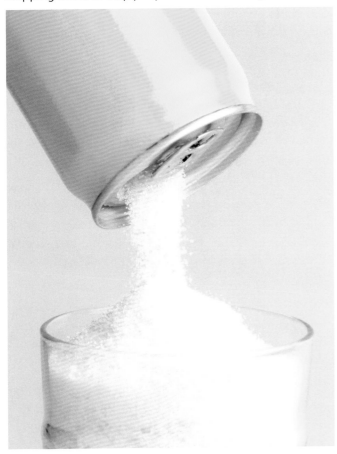

Dr Ian Johnson, nutrition researcher and emeritus fellow at the Quadram Institute in Norfolk, said: 'This new guideline is based on a thorough assessment of the latest scientific literature and it emphasises that the use of artificial sweeteners is not a good strategy for achieving weight loss by reducing dietary energy intake.

'However, this should not be interpreted as an indication that sugar intake has no relevance to weight control.

'A better alternative to the use of artificial sweeteners is to reduce consumption of manufactured products containing free sugars, such as sugar-sweetened beverages, to use raw or lightly processed fruit as a source of sweetness, and perhaps, in the longer term, to try to reduce one's overall taste for sweetness.'

An International Sweeteners Association spokesperson said: 'Low/no calorie sweeteners are one of the most thoroughly researched ingredients in the world and continue to be a helpful tool to manage obesity, diabetes and dental diseases.

'They offer consumers an alternative to reduce sugar and calorie intake with the sweet taste they know and expect.

'There has been an overwhelming amount of scientific literature supporting low/no calorie sweeteners' utility for weight management, including the WHO-commissioned systematic review itself.

'The International Sweeteners Association believes it is a disservice to not recognise the public health benefits of low/no calorie sweeteners and is disappointed that the WHO's conclusions are largely based on low certainty evidence from observational studies, which are at high risk of reverse causality.'

NSS approved for use in the UK include acesulfame K, aspartame, erythritol, saccharin, sorbitol, steviol glycosides, sucralose and xylitol.

16 May 2023

Research

Do some research on natural alternatives to sugar and sweeteners. What can be used instead?

Consider...

How do you think you can reduce your taste for sweetness?

Can you wean yourself off of sugar?

Write some changes that you can make to reduce how much sugar and sweeteners you have in your diet.

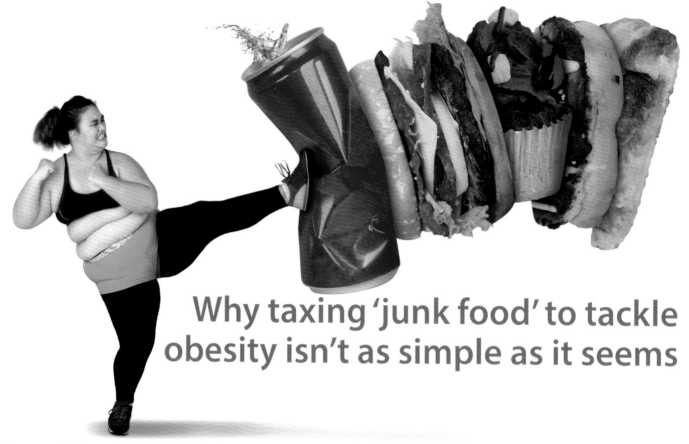

Why taxing 'junk food' to tackle obesity isn't as simple as it seems

An article from The Conversation.

By Duane Mellor, Lead for Evidence-Based Medicine and Nutrition, Aston Medical School, Aston University

Former prime minister Tony Blair has called for more taxes on junk food to tackle the UK's obesity crisis. This includes extending sugar taxes beyond just soft drinks, as well as taxing food that is high in salt and fat. Blair also called for restrictions on advertising unhealthy food.

The former PM believes this is the only way to save the NHS. 'We've got to shift from a service that's treating people when they're ill to a service that is focused on wellbeing, on prevention, on how people live more healthy lives,' he told The Times Health Commission.

But is it as simple as that? A levy on sugary drinks was introduced in the UK in 2018 which led to drinks makers reformulating their products so they contained less sugar. A year later, the British public was consuming less sugar. However, sugar consumption had been falling in Britain before the levy was introduced. Once this was factored into the analysis, there was no significant fall in sugar consumption.

Denmark experimented with a fat tax and it had similar underwhelming results. It was hailed as a world-leading public health policy when it was introduced in October 2011 but was abandoned 15 months later.

According to one survey, only 7% of Danes reduced the amount of butter, cream and cheese they bought. A different survey found that 80% did not change their food shopping habits at all.

However, whether or not levies on unhealthy food work is difficult to determine. Advocates for these programmes tend to highlight positive effects based on data modelling rather than actual changes in people's weight and health. Detractors, on the other hand, quickly challenge such policies as being the enactment of the 'nanny state'.

Where and what to tax?

Although the UK's sugar tax led to drinks being reformulated to have less sugar, it also had some unintended consequences. For example, sugary drinks called slushies needed to have glycerol (E422) added to them to maintain their slush (artificial sweeteners failed to produce the required 'slush').

While this is safe for most older children and adults, the Food Standards Agency identified a possible risk of glycerol intoxication in smaller children and suggested sales should be restricted to children five years old and older.

Another unintended consequence is making the poor poorer by raising the price of food. If taxes or levies are extended beyond drinks and sugar to include all food high in fat, salt and sugar, the cost of this reformulation is likely to be passed on to the consumer.

With the current cost of living crisis, this is simply not acceptable to politicians or many of the public. If such levies are introduced, they need to be a smarter version of the soft drinks industry levy. It should drive food producers to change the food they produce, making less healthy ingredients cost more while making it more profitable to grow and supply healthier food.

What is 'junk' food?

The next challenge is to identify which food to tax.

Blair suggested 'junk food', which he defined as high in fat, salt and sugar - often called HFSS foods. It is these foods that can no longer be advertised on Transport for London sites.

This has been hailed as a success. These restrictions on advertising are estimated to have significantly decreased the average amount of HFSS foods households buy each week.

This data was then used to claim that this change reduced the number of people with obesity by 100,000. This claim has been heavily criticised. It is an estimate, and the change in the number of people who are overweight or obese linked to the advertising ban is unknown.

So, although there may be some merit in tackling advertising, it perhaps needs to be smarter and respond to modern and emerging trends in advertising strategies. The focus on out-of-home advertising, which is the Transport for London approach, does not look at how social media and online advertising linked to cookies and trackers can build a message for potential consumers. Challenging how advertisers link campaigns across media is probably more effective.

An alternative is to focus where advertising is permitted. For example, regulating billboards near schools so that they only show healthy messages may be a more effective solution.

This is before considering the potentially stigmatising language in calling food 'junk' food, especially given the message is focused on helping poorer people. Perhaps this is why there has been a move to use terms such as 'ultra-processed food'.

Both, however, are slightly subjective. The HFSS definition could include cheese and Greek yoghurt and therefore might suggest that these foods receive an advertising ban. Whereas a fast-food meal with water and carrot sticks – although these may be the least popular meal option – can still be advertised.

When promoting healthier dietary choices, we need to make options like vegetables attractive. This can be difficult for people on low incomes, who might avoid trying new food that might be rejected and wasted. Instead, go for family favourites which might be less healthy but will make sure everyone is full within their budget.

So what are the answers? Perhaps not top-down approaches, such as those proposed by Blair. An example of how our food system can be changed has been set out in the Birmingham Food System Strategy. This sets out how small local food businesses make healthier food widely available across the city, as well as provide employment in the city. This sets out a community-led approach that encourages a city-wide food supply that is healthy for people and the planet.

To solve a complex problem you need subtle and connected changes in many areas that are designed with and are acceptable to those with the most to gain, but who are struggling on low incomes.

15 September 2023

Debate

As a class, debate a taxation on food high in sugar, salt and fat. One half of the class will be for the new tax and the rest will be against.

Consider what the effects of the tax would be, and how any money raised could be spent.

Write

Write a persuasive letter to your MP on banning advertising of 'Junk' food. Give your reasons and provide why you think that the ban would be a good idea.

THE C⭕NVERSATION

The fight against ultra-processed foods and food labelling loopholes!

By Vandana Chatlani, BANT Registered Nutritionist® NT Dip, mBANT, rCNHC

Reducing obesity and metabolic disease depends on a return to real food and a culture of nutritious eating. Reading ingredient labels and avoiding marketing traps can empower us to make healthier choices.

But can we escape the junk food cycle?

More than 50% of foods consumed in the UK are ultra-processed according to research. These include packaged breads, breakfast cereals, reconstituted meat products, ready meals, confectionery, biscuits, cakes, pastries, industrial chips, soft drinks and fruit juices.

Our current food climate is dominated by ultra-processed foods which fuel metabolic dysregulation through their high fat, salt and sugar content (HFSS). These are pushed by BIG Food; multinational conglomerates that monopolise food production and distribution putting profit ahead of consumer health and wellbeing. As a nation, the UK has become addicted to sickly sweetened food and drinks and highly processed foods that, let's face it, aren't really foods at all. Manufacturers are exploiting legal loopholes, an absence of regulation and a lack of political will to fuel the soaring consumption of these products to the detriment of our health. These foods are easy to come by and cheap to buy, but their risks to our health are costly both in personal terms and to the NHS as a whole. Ultra-processed foods have consistently been linked with increased levels of obesity, diabetes, weight gain and other non-communicable diseases.

More than 4 billion people could be overweight or obese by 2035, compared with 2.6 billion in 2020 according to a report published by the World Obesity Federation.

The statistics in the UK are equally alarming. Almost three quarters of people aged 45-74 in England are overweight or obese according to The Health Survey for England 2021 published late last year. Overall numbers show that 68.6% of men and 59% of women are either overweight or obese.

In Scotland, figures from 2021 put 31% of adults in the obese category and 36% in the overweight category, while in Wales in the same year 26% of women and 23% of men reported being obese.

Our children are inheriting the poor eating patterns that have become so pervasive in adults who are lured in by clever marketing to consume processed convenience food that are calorific and void of nutrients. This has contributed to 23.4% of 10-11-year-olds in England being obese and 14.3% being overweight according to data from the National Child Measurement Programme published by NHS Digital.

The problem is exacerbated in the most deprived areas of England where prevalence of obesity or being overweight is 9 percentage points higher than in the least deprived areas of the country. Moreover, people from black ethnic groups have been shown to have the highest rates of excess weight with 72% of adults from these groups classified as overweight or living with obesity in the year ending November 2021 – the highest percentage out of all ethnic groups.

In lower income countries and communities, a preference towards highly processed foods is a major factor in increasing rates of obesity. Figures estimate that access to healthy food is unaffordable for almost 3.1 billion people worldwide. Our agrifood systems have evolved today so that the cost of a healthy diet is five times greater than the cost of diets that meet our energy requirements only through a staple cereal. Low-priced foods high in energy and low in nutritional value are on the rise. And this trend has led to an increase in associated health risks linked to mortality and diseases such as diabetes, obesity and overweight. Statistics indicate that between 702 and 828 million people were affected by hunger in 2021. On the other hand, numbers in 2022 show that more than one billion people are obese and by 2025, around 167 million people – adults and children – will become less healthy because they are overweight or obese.

The world's food systems are out of kilter and imbalanced. They have not been designed to meet our dietary needs, but instead focus on business gains. As the cost-of-living crisis rages on and many struggle to make ends meet, food choices depend largely if not solely on affordability. The cycle becomes a vicious one as eating low-cost often means consuming calorific, processed foods packed with additives and lacking in vitamins and minerals. Inevitably then, those who are already financially burdened, are saddled with the health consequences of consuming products that companies know very well lead to overweight and obesity, hypertension, metabolic syndrome, cardiovascular diseases, and gastrointestinal disorders .

Understanding the processing spectrum

As supermarkets lure us in with clever marketing strategies, brightly coloured packaging and dubious health claims, it has become more important than ever for us to understand our food and how it is processed.

The NOVA international classification system, developed by Carlos Monteiro and his team at the Center for Epidemiological Research in Nutrition and Health at the University of São Paulo in Brazil, provides a useful starting point to understand different levels of food processing.

In reality, processed foods are designed to increase flavour, extend shelf-life, and ensure transportability, all of which reduce nutritional quality.

It is vital to recognise that there are varying levels of food processing. Because most of us no longer live in agrarian settings, most of our food tends to be processed to some degree.

Unprocessed foods or those that are minimally processed are those that may have been roasted, boiled, ground, dried, crushed, fermented or made easier to eat for example by removing inedible or unwanted parts. For example, spiralized courgettes or 'courgetti', frozen blueberries, walnuts (with their shells removed), and salmon which has been descaled and filleted. Generally speaking, these processes do not rely on the addition of salt, sugar, fats, additives, etc., and instead focus on making the food more convenient to use, long-lasting and/or diverse.

You then have processed culinary ingredients such as butter, sugar, salt, condiments and oils that may be dried, pressed, ground, milled and refined to season and cook foods in the unprocessed fresh food category to enhance flavour. These ingredients – think paprika, olive oil, cream, and maple syrup – are not meant to be eaten on their own.

Processed foods such as tinned sardines, canned chickpeas, baked beans, camembert and focaccia, for example, often combine oil, salt, sugar or the substances from the second group of culinary ingredients, with foods from the unprocessed or minimally processed group. These foods may be cooked, baked, preserved or fermented without alcohol to increase their durability or enhance their appearance, smell and taste.

Ultra-processed foods, by contrast, are modified to such an extent through multiple types of processing that they barely resemble the fresh or minimally processed items in the first group. These foods and drinks such as chicken nuggets, ice-cream, instant noodles, vegetarian burgers, cheese twists, tortilla wraps, bourbon biscuits, breakfast cereals, margarine, instant soups, sausage rolls, cakes, ready meals and soft drinks, often include salt, sugar, oils and fats, as well as other ingredients and additives like lactose, emulsifiers, gluten, hydrolysed proteins, high-fructose corn syrup, and artificial colours and flavourings. These ingredients have undergone significant processing themselves. Many of these additives are found only in ultra-processed foods in order to mask unpleasant tastes or enhance the appearance, attractiveness and flavour of the final product.

Because many ultra-processed foods contain so little real food, one can understand why they lack any nutrient density. But the problem doesn't stop there. Not only are these foods lacking in vitamins, minerals, healthy protein, fibre and more, their high levels of salt, sugar, oils, fats and additives makes them addictive – so we end up consuming more empty calories because these foods don't satiate us like whole foods do.

What are the consequences of a diet dominated by ultra-processed foods? Studies have shown associations between such foods and obesity, weight gain, cardio-metabolic risks, cancer, type-2 diabetes, irritable bowel syndrome and depression. Among kids, the effects include obesity, weight gain, cardio-metabolic risks and asthma.

Food labels: The devil is in the detail

So what can we do to avoid the processed food trap?

Reading food labels carefully may be one way to reduce our reliance on foods filled with artificial flavourings, colours and ingredients.

Food labelling is strictly governed by law in the UK and so false, misleading descriptions are illegal. Manufacturers can only make statements about their foods if they are accurate. For example, companies cannot label a product 'reduced calorie' unless it is much lower in calories than the regular version.

Manufacturers are mandated to show the country of origin if customers might be misled without this information, for example, if the label for a packet of paneer shows the Taj Mahal, but the paneer is made in the UK.

Group 1 Unprocessed or minimally processed foods	**Group 2** Processed culinary ingredients	**Group 3** Processed foods	**Group 4** Ultra-processed foods
Fresh, dry, or frozen vegetables or fruit, grains, legumes, meat, fish, eggs, nuts and seeds.	Plant oils (e.g. olive oil, coconut oil), animal fats (e.g. cream, butter, lard), maple syrup, sugar, honey and salt.	Canned/pickled vegetables, meat, fish or fruit, artisanal bread, cheese, salted meats, wine, beer and cider.	Sugar sweetened beverages, sweet and savoury packaged snacks, reconstituted meat products, pre-prepared frozen dishes, canned/instant soups, chicken nuggets, ice cream.
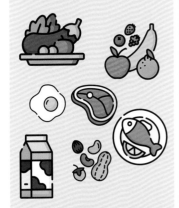	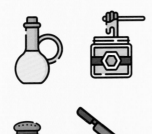	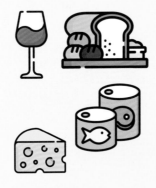	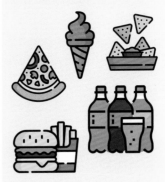
Processing includes removal of inedible/unwanted parts. Does not add substances to the original food.	Substances derived from Group 1 foods or from nature by processes including pressing, refining, grinding, milling and drying.	Processing of foods from Group 1 or 2 with the addition of oil, salt, or sugar by means of canning, pickling, smoking, curing or fermentation.	Formulations made from a series of processes including extraction and chemical modification. Includes very little intact Group 1 foods.

Increasing level of processing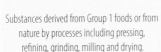

Source: British Association for Nutrition and Lifestyle Medicine (BANT).
Image credit: Spectrum of processing of foods based on the NOVA classification. The figure provides examples of foods and types of processing methods within each NOVA classification group. Definitions are adapted from Monteiro et al. (2018).

If the primary ingredient in the food comes from a place that is different to where the product says it was made, the label must show this. For example, a pork pie labelled 'British' that is produced in the UK with pork from Germany, must state 'with pork from Germany' or 'made with pork from outside the UK'.

Foods must indicate if they have undergone any processing, for example, 'smoked' salmon, 'dried' cherries, or 'shredded, pickled' beetroot.

Every ingredient must be listed on labels for foods which contain two or more ingredients. Ingredients must be listed in order of weight, with the main ingredient first. Companies are also expected to show the percentage of an ingredient if it is highlighted by the labelling or a picture on a package, for example 'extra cheese', mentioned in a 'cheese and onion pasty', or a food normally connected with its name by consumers, for example, fruit in a summer pudding.

Images on food packaging must also be accurate. So, a pot of blueberry yoghurt which contains artificial flavouring rather than real fruit, is not permitted to have a picture of blueberries on the pot (although manufacturers have gotten away with cartoon blueberries before).

Food packaging must show an appropriate warning on the label if the food contains certain ingredients. For example, if the food contains artificial colours such as 'allura red (E129)', 'carmoisine (E122)', or 'quinoline yellow (E104)', the label should state 'may have an adverse effect on activity and attention in children'.

Exploiting legal loopholes & the bitter truth about sugar

Food labels are intended to protect and inform consumers, but many can be misleading. Sadly, our quest to select foods with more vitamins, minerals and fibre, and less trans-fat, cholesterol, and salt, is not always a straightforward one. Navigating food labels can be a minefield.

Assessing healthiness based on labels can be tricky. Positive labels such as 'natural', 'organic', and 'low-fat' can be deceiving in terms of the benefits they confer. Some data, such as the content of 'free sugars', i.e. the sugar that is added to a product rather than the sugar that appears naturally in a piece of fruit, for example, is not legally required to appear on a label.

Instead, products must show 'total sugars' which include both naturally occurring sugars and added sugars. This makes it difficult for consumers to know how much added sugar they are consuming. For example, full-fat fresh milk contains 9.4g of total sugars per serving (200ml), but none of these are 'free sugars' as they all come naturally from the milk. In comparison, a brand of chocolate milk shows the same number of total sugars – 9.4g per 200ml – but upon closer inspection of the ingredients, this includes a sweetener, sucralose, and rice starch which breaks down into sugar.

Appreciating how sugars and starches are highlighted on food labels is vital if we are to make healthier choices.

For example, despite having a very high glycaemic index (GI), refined starches such as maltodextrin, which can be found in many processed foods such as pasta, cereals, salad dressings and sweets, do not have to be labelled as sugars. In fact, maltodextrin is excluded in the definition of sugar used for nutrition labelling. High GI foods are rapidly absorbed into our bloodstream and lead to sugar spikes, and excess sugar is often a major culprit for obesity and type 2 diabetes.

Fructose is another problematic ingredient. It occurs naturally in fruit and honey but is also used as a free sugar in confectionery and sugary drinks. Food manufacturers can include a health claim on their products stating that the consumption of foods containing fructose leads to a lower blood glucose rise compared to foods containing sucrose or glucose. This is if the fructose used reduces the content of sucrose or glucose by 30%.

But despite the truth that fructose has a lower GI than sucrose and glucose, consuming high amounts can affect our liver and compromise the function of our hunger and satiety hormones, leptin and ghrelin, so we think we are still hungry and end up overeating. Unlike glucose, which can be metabolised by all of our cells, fructose can only be broken down by our liver. High fructose consumption has been associated with non-alcoholic fatty liver disease, insulin resistance and diabetes, and obesity. So the suggestion that fructose is a healthy sugar alternative is too simplistic and misleading. The fact is, fructose is taxed like other sugars, so why are companies allowed to attach a positive health claim to it being a good substitute for sucrose?

All carbohydrate foods including grains, fruits, cereals, dairy and starchy vegetables contain sugars. In the case of whole foods, some of these sugars are bound to other nutrients, such as fibre, fat and protein, which help slow their release into the bloodstream and thus reduce the sugar highs and subsequent dramatic crashes that we experience. Avoiding 'free sugars' – the ones added to products like fizzy drinks, sweets, yoghurts, sauces and breakfast cereals, we can maintain balanced energy levels and a healthy weight.

Since 2018, the UK has taxed drinks which contain 5g or more free sugar per 100ml. The levy saw a fall of 35.4% in total sugar sold in soft drinks between 2015 and 2019. However, despite this, obesity levels have continued to rise, suggesting that the government needs to enact tougher policies to push food companies towards healthier and more sustainable manufacturing practices.

The way forward: how to make healthier choices.

In March, the British Association of Nutritional and Lifestyle Medicine supported the resignation of Henry Dimbleby from his role as government food adviser in protest at the government's inaction against obesity and junk food culture. BANT has continuously advocated for stronger policies to tackle the obesity epidemic.

Prior to stepping down from his role, Dimbleby published the National Food Strategy, an independent review for government aimed at reshaping our food system so that it is stable, safe, sustainable, affordable and nutritious. Dimbleby's recommendations include the following:

* Introduce a sugar and salt reformulation tax and use some of the revenue to help get fresh fruit and vegetables to low-income families

Eat a **rainbow**
7 a day
(5 veg and 2 fruit)

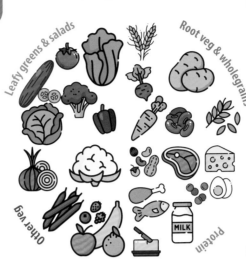

Health & wellbeing
Sleeping and feeding times are important determinants of overall health. Sleep 7-9 hours, ideally starting before midnight. Eat regular meals and advoid snacking.

Salads & vegetables
Unlimited salads, leafy greens and vegetables, excluding root vegetables.

Drinks
Drink water, tea (black, green, fruit and herbal infusions), avoid drinks that are high in sugar or artificial sweeteners including fruit juice.

Fruit
Eat 1-3 palm-sized portions of fruit a day. Berries in abundance and local and seasonal fruit.

Multi-vitamin and extra vitamin D for most people. Probiotics and blood sugar support, as advised by nutrition healthcare professionals.

Leafy greens & salads

Root veg & wholegrains

Other veg

Protein

MILK

Exercise
Keep moving and stay active. Use the stairs, walk whenever you can. Walk an extra stop. Park further away. Stand rather tha sit at your desk.

Eat root vegetables as well as wholegrains (like wild and brown rice, whole oats, quinoa). Limit refined grains (like pasta and bread) which affect the body in a similar way to sugar.

Oils
Use olive oil as your everyday fat for both cooking and seasoning, and butter in moderation. Avoid margarines and trans fats. Eat raw nuts, seeds and avocados.

Make fish, poultry and eggs your principal sources of protein, and eat lean red meat, bacon and other processed meats only occasionally. Eat pulses (lentils, beans, chickpeas) and nuts and seeds as vegetable protein. Limit dairy to a small matchbox of cheese, half a cup of live unsweetened yoghurt or a small glass of milk a day.

The wellness solution

Source: British Association for Nutrition and Lifestyle Medicine (BANT)

- Introduce mandatory reporting for large food companies
- Invest £1 billion in innovation to create a better food system
- Strengthen government procurement rules to ensure that taxpayer money is spent on healthy and sustainable food.

Without adequate government support and the influence of powerful food manufacturers whose profit lines are prioritised ahead of consumer wellbeing, navigating a healthy diet and knowing what to eat has become more challenging than ever before.

The food and drink industry is the UK's largest manufacturing sector, surpassing economic contributions from the automotive and aerospace manufacturing industries. In 2022, total business investment in the industry amounted to £4 billion, up by 7.9% from 2020. With such power, BIG Food has the potential to transform consumer health, reduce chronic disease and sustain a more productive population. Conscientious, science-backed policies are the need of the hour.

But there is a lack of political will to bring about meaningful change. The government has failed to do its part to tackle obesity and associated chronic conditions by delaying restrictions on junk food promotions and advertising to children, and refusing to tax manufacturers on the sugar they add in processed food.

So, what can we do?

Thankfully, there are several shopping strategies we can adopt to rid ourselves of the ultra-processed food trap.

Better awareness of food labels is crucial starting point to identify and reduce the amount of processed and ultra-processed food we consume.

One indicator of a processed product will be its never-ending list of ingredients, many of which seem unrecognisable or impossible to find in natural form. In most cases, less is more. Take butter, for example. The sole ingredient in one brand of organic butter is cow's milk. Compare this with a brand of margarine, which has the following: water, vegetable oils in varying proportions (palm oil, rapeseed oil), reconstituted buttermilk, salt, emulsifier: mono- and diglycerides of fatty acids; preservative: potassium sorbate; acidity regulator: lactic acid; vitamin E, flavouring, colour: carotenes; vitamin A and vitamin D. Which would you pick?

Keep an eye out for additives and avoid foods with these ingredients as much as possible. Additives include artificial colours and dyes, artificial flavours and flavour enhancers and non-sugar sweeteners. It's also worth taking stock of processing terms. So foods and drinks which indicate that they have been 'carbonated', or include 'bulking', 'anti-caking', and 'glazing' agents, for example, should be avoided.

When shopping, stay away from products which include 'free sugars' such as fructose, high-fructose corn syrup, fruit juice concentrate, cane sugar, crystalline sucrose, glucose and honey. Honey is often perceived as a healthier sugar, because of its potential anti-inflammatory and anti-bacterial properties. But it is also high in fructose and is absorbed in the same way as other sugars, so it is important to consume in moderation.

Steer clear of buy-one-get-one-free deals, which are often applied to junk foods. These deals persuade us to buy more than we need, resulting in excessive calories or resulting in food waste when these foods cannot be finished.

The traffic light system gives us some indication of which foods may be healthy, but it has its limitations. Look deeper

White	**Yellow**	**Orange**	**Red**	**Blue-Purple**	**Green**
Cauliflower	Bell peppers	Apricots	Blood orange	Aubergine	Broccoli
Garlic	Corn	Butternut squash	Cherries	Beetroot	Celery
Ginger	Lemon	Carrots	Cranberries	Blackberries	Cucumber
Mushrooms	Apples	Nectarine	Pomegranates	Blueberries	Green beans
Onions	Spaghetti squash	Orange	Radishes	Figs	Green peppers
Soya	Starfruit	Sweet potato	Red cabbage	Plums	Leafy greens

Eat a **rainbow** every day

A diverse selection of plant foods optimises your phytonutrients intake

Source: British Association for Nutrition and Lifestyle Medicine (BANT)

at the list of ingredients and you'll see the traffic light only reveals so much about food composition and nutrient density. So don't rely solely on the green light when choosing what to put in your basket.

Let's look at tortilla wraps. They contain only 1.5g of sugar per wrap, and so they get a green light in this category (while fat, saturated fat and salt all come under the amber light). Does that mean tortillas are a fairly nutritious choice? Let's scan the ingredients: fortified British wheat flour (wheat flour, calcium carbonate, niacin, iron, thiamin), water, palm oil, humectant: glycerol; raising agents: disodium diphosphate, sodium hydrogen carbonate; sugar, acidity regulator: citric acid; emulsifier: mono- and diglycerides of fatty acids; preservative: calcium propionate; salt, wheat starch, flour treatment agent: l-cysteine. Does that seem healthy? Should our daily bread require so many ingredients?

How about batch cooking and freezing our own tortillas for easy access? A recipe for homemade flour tortillas uses flour, baking powder, salt, olive oil and water. Don't those real food ingredients seem so simple and appealing?

Be savvy about marketing traps. The word 'natural', for instance, evokes a sense of healthy, unprocessed food. The Food Standards Agency states that 'natural' should mean that the food is made up of ingredients produced by nature. But many foods contain chemicals renamed to be more appealing to consumers. 'Carrot concentrate', for example, is a highly processed ingredient that is used to give foods a bright yellow hue.

Organic food is certainly better for you from the point of view that it is free from harmful pesticides. However, just because something is certified organic does not mean it is nutritious, as this simply indicates how the food is produced. Organic foods can be high in saturated fat and sugar.

Similarly, 'plant-based' is often synonymous with healthiness (and climate consciousness), however, many plant-based items such as meat substitutes, can be highly processed, high in fat, salt and sugar.

Foods that claim to be 'low sugar' can still be calorific as well as high in fat. The label 'no added sugar' can be misleading too, as manufacturers can use fruit juice concentrate as a sweetener which does not have to be labelled as 'added sugar'.

'Low fat' foods indicate that a food has less than 3g of fat per 100g. However, it is common for food producers to substitute the eliminated fat with sugar to maintain flavour.

One of the best things we can do for ourselves is return to a culture of whole foods and home-cooking. Instead of perusing the endless aisles of packaged food in your supermarket, spend some time in the fresh fruit, veg, meat and fish sections. We lead busy lives, so sometimes relying on some minimally processed foods like a stir fry mix with beansprouts peppers, sweetcorn, cabbage, carrot and onions is our best bet.

Read those labels and keep things simple. Look out for seasonal produce to bring colour and variety to your table while saving costs. Think brussel sprouts in the winter, rhubarb in early spring, wild nettles in the summer and pumpkins in autumn.

Fill your basket with colour and meal plan so you get the most out of your fresh produce. A tray of roasted vegetables works beautifully with a piece of roasted chicken and leftovers can be eaten for lunch the next day. Build hearty stews or daals with vegetables, lentils, herbs and spices. Create deliciously cool salads with crisp apples, walnuts and pomegranates. Take inspiration from different cuisines and play around with ingredients to maximise vitamin and mineral diversity.

28 June 2023

Portion size: cause and solution to overweight and obesity?

Getting portion sizes right is an important part of a healthy and balanced diet.

By Professor Eric Robinson, University of Liverpool

Getting portion sizes right is an important part of a healthy and balanced diet.

The causes of obesity are complex, but overconsumption of food and sugary drinks is a key direct determinant, driven in part by large portion sizes. Recent research conducted at the University of Liverpool suggests that portion sizes may not only contribute to overweight and obesity but also may be part of the possible solution.

Survey data estimates that between 1980 and 2019, the prevalence of obesity in England increased from 6% to 27% in men and 9% to 29% in women. At the same time portion sizes of many foods served at home and out of the home have increased, pointing to the possibility that larger portions may have played a contributory role in rising obesity.

To tease apart what kind of impact this is likely to have had on diets several studies have examined the relationship between portion size and the amount people eat at meals. A 2016 review concluded that portion sizes that are twice as large as usual increase meal consumption by more than a third (35%). Whilst these studies show a clear effect of portion size on intake at a single eating occasion, what they don't tell us is whether the impact portion size has is maintained over time and how it influences body weight. For example, although a larger portion at lunch may increase calorie intake for lunch, maybe later in the day your body naturally compensates for this by requiring less food to feel full. If this was the case, then it could also mean that reducing portion sizes may not be useful for weight management because any reductions in portion size would be made up for later in the day. In our current food environment where energy dense foods are easily accessible, it is also important to consider what happens when large portions are continually available. Will people keep overeating, or will compensatory mechanisms sense the accumulating excess energy and limit intake?

The only way to answer this question is to look at experiments in which participants have been randomly allocated to be served smaller vs. larger portions over time and then their daily energy intake or body weight has been measured.

This is what researchers from the department of psychology at the University of Liverpool did in a new piece of research. In the systematic review, they looked at studies that had manipulated portion sizes and measured energy intake across the course of a minimum of one day. What's important to note about these studies is that if participants did want to make up for or 'compensate' for the smaller portions provided, they had opportunities to do so throughout the study day/s. The researchers analysed data from 14 studies and found that portion size does have a prolonged effect on what people eat – smaller portions at breakfast, lunch or evening meals result in people eating fewer calories (approximately 235 kcal on average) daily. The other key finding was from a smaller subset of studies which looked at changes in body weight. Participants served smaller portions gained 0.6kg less weight than those served larger portions which suggests that getting portion sizes right could help with preventing weight gain and managing weight loss.

But is it as simple as reducing your portion sizes of all foods and meals? We think not! The amount (volume) of food we eat does impact how full we feel and therefore the likely best portion size orientated solution for weight management is to be tactical – decrease the portion size of more energy dense foods and serve generous portion sizes of much lower calorie foods (e.g. vegetables). This approach could be particularly valuable for weight management as it should help people manage the number of calories being consumed at meals without feeling constantly hungry. The British Nutrition Foundation looks at this concept in their information on the energy density approach. It's also in keeping with the British Nutrition Foundation's recently revised *Get portion wise!* resource which has lots of practical tips and advice on getting portion sizes right.

2022

Key Facts

- Survey data estimates that between 1980 and 2019, the prevalence of obesity in England increased from 6% to 27% in men and 9% to 29% in women.

- Smaller portions at breakfast, lunch or evening meals result in people eating fewer calories (approximately 235 kcal on average) daily.

Research

Have a look at the *Get portion wise!* resource. Do any of the portion sizes surprise you? Are they bigger or smaller than you expected?

www.nutrition.org.uk

Your balanced diet – get portion wise!

Why think about portion size?

Most of us probably do not think about portion size when we eat – it depends on what we would usually have, how hungry we feel and how much is in a pack or on a plate. But having a healthy, balanced diet is about getting the right types of foods and drinks in the right amounts. These guides aim to help you find the right balance for you – it's not only about how much you eat, it's also about eating differently!

The portion sizes given are not government recommendations but suggestions of practical portion sizes for healthy adults for a range of foods and drinks. These can be used to complement the government's Eatwell Guide, which provides guidance on the proportions of the food groups that make up a healthy, balanced diet.

Getting portion size right for you

We're all individuals with different needs. For healthy adults the types of different foods and drinks we need are pretty much the same for all of us. But, the amount of food we need varies from person to person.

The portion sizes we give are averages for healthy adults, based on a daily calorie need of 2000kcal – the amount estimated for an average, adult woman. If you're tall or very active you may need more. If you're a small person or are trying to lose weight, you may need smaller portions. If you use the hand measures we give, portion sizes will vary with the size of your hands and so, generally, bigger people will get bigger portions and smaller people will get smaller portions.

There are lots of different ways to eat a healthy, balanced diet and you can use this guidance to fit in with your preferences and beliefs – from a flexitarian (plenty of plant-based foods with some animal foods), to a vegetarian or vegan diet. It's about balancing the food groups and finding the portion sizes that are right for you.

Each day, aim for:

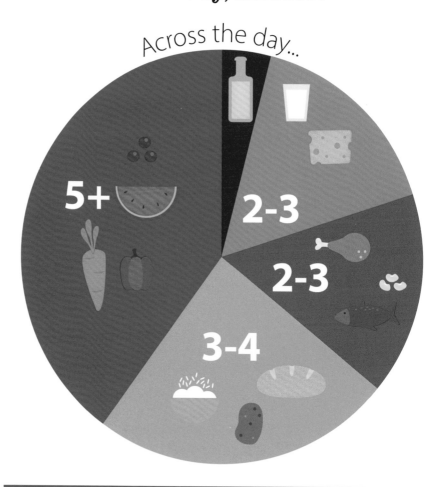

Across the day...

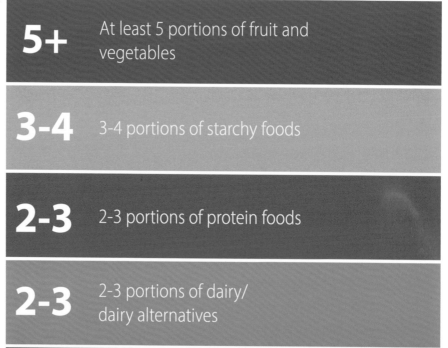

5+	At least 5 portions of fruit and vegetables
3-4	3-4 portions of starchy foods
2-3	2-3 portions of protein foods
2-3	2-3 portions of dairy/ dairy alternatives
Small amounts	Small amounts of unsaturated oils and spreads

Source: British Nutrition Foundation

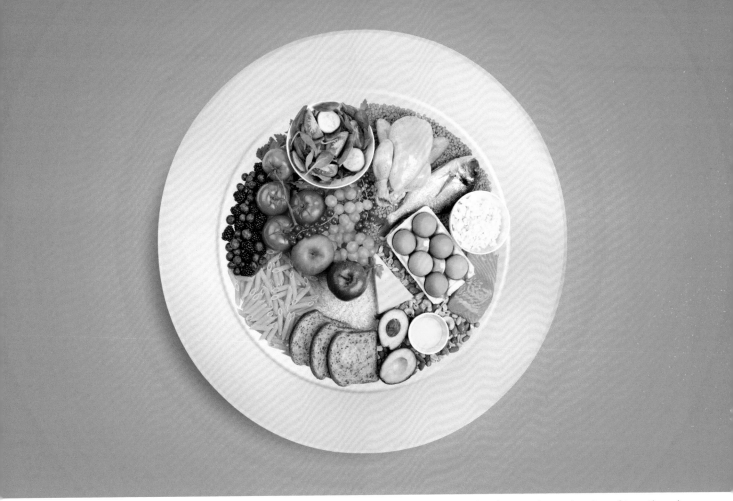

Across the day

From each food group we are suggesting:

- Fruit and vegetables: 5+ portions per day

- Starchy carbohydrates: 3-4 portions per day

- Beans, pulses, fish, eggs, meat and other proteins: 2-3 portions per day

- Dairy and alternatives: 2-3 portions per day

Measuring portion size

If you really want to measure portion size accurately the best way is to weigh your food but we have provided some practical measures using your hands and spoons that you can use to get an idea of sensible portion sizes.

For example:

- Two handfuls of dried pasta shapes or rice (75g)

- A bunch of spaghetti the size of a £1 coin, measured using your finger and thumb (75g)

- The amount of cooked pasta or rice that would fit in two hands cupped together (180g)

- A baked potato about the size of your fist (220g)

- About three handfuls of breakfast cereal (40g)

- A piece of grilled chicken breast about size of your whole hand (120g)

- A piece of cheddar cheese about the size of two thumbs together (30g)

- About one tablespoon of peanut butter (20g)

- About three teaspoons of soft cheese (30g)

We first published these guides in 2019 and in 2021 we have been working to evaluate the originals. We have talked to a range of different people through in-home interviews, online surveys an industry panel and a consumer panel, to see if they found the guides useful to help them eat a more balanced diet. The *Your balanced diet – get portion wise* guides have been updated to make the key messages clearer and to include more information about how to put the advice into practice in meals and snacks. We have also updated some of the portion size measures in the full portion size guide and added more foods to the lists.

We hope these guides help you put a healthy, balanced diet into practice and to find your balance!

Please visit: www.nutrition.org.uk to download the guides.

November 2021

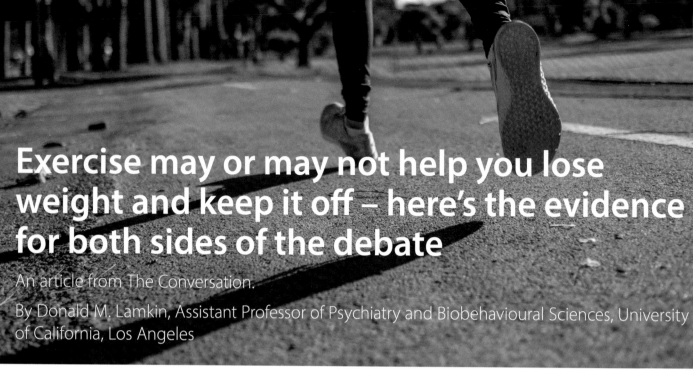

Exercise may or may not help you lose weight and keep it off – here's the evidence for both sides of the debate

An article from The Conversation.

By Donald M. Lamkin, Assistant Professor of Psychiatry and Biobehavioural Sciences, University of California, Los Angeles

The global fitness industry will generate over US$80 billion in revenue in 2023, estimates suggest. And why not, given the many excellent reasons to exercise? Better cardiovascular health, lower risk of Type 2 diabetes, stronger immune system – the list goes on.

One of the biggest reasons many people choose to exercise is to lose weight. As a biobehavioural scientist, I study links between behaviour and health, and I heed the time-honoured advice that eating less and exercising more are necessary to lose weight. But a recent debate in the scientific community highlights the growing suspicion that the 'exercising more' part of this advice may be erroneous.

At the centre of the debate is the constrained total energy expenditure hypothesis, which asserts that exercise won't help you burn more calories overall because your body will compensate by burning fewer calories after your workout. Thus, exercise won't help you lose weight even if it will benefit your health in countless other ways.

Obesity researchers take issue with this hypothesis, because it's based on observational research rather than randomised controlled trials, or RCTs, the gold standard of scientific evidence. In RCTs, participants are randomly assigned to either a treatment or a control group, which allows researchers to determine whether the treatment causes an effect. Randomised controlled trials have shown that exercise causes weight loss.

What the evidence says

Spectators of this hypothesis have emphasized the importance of systematically reviewing the evidence from all gold-standard trials. They pointed to a 2021 review of more than 100 exercise studies that examined the effect on weight loss in adults of aerobic, resistance or high-intensity interval training in combination or alone. The review concluded that supervised exercise regimens do cause weight loss, even if only a modest amount.

So that settles the debate, yes? If you eat too much dessert, then you can just go on an extra run to burn off those extra calories, right?

Well, not exactly.

If extra physical exertion burns extra calories overall, then exercise should also keep the weight from coming back after low-calorie dieting. But keeping those lost pounds off after dieting is a common challenge. The same 2021 review includes the few randomised controlled trials that address the question of whether exercise facilitates weight maintenance. However, the results weren't as good as they were for weight loss. The researchers found that six to 12 months of aerobic exercise, resistance training or both after dieting did not prevent weight regain in adults.

Exercise adherence

But what about compliance? Did all the people in those studies actually exercise regularly?

The 2021 review found only one randomised controlled trial on weight maintenance that reported an objective compliance rate, meaning each exercise session was supervised by a trainer. This tells us the percentage of time that participants in the study actually exercised as prescribed.

In that trial, the compliance rate was only 64% for 25 post-menopausal women who completed a resistance training program after diet-induced weight loss. This was for a regimen in which participants had to come in and exercise two to three times per week for an entire year. From the perspective of keeping up with a program for that long, doing so 64% of the time doesn't seem so bad.

But they still gained back as much weight as the 29 women in the control group who were not enrolled in the exercise program.

Energy balance

Many people would say that it's all about balancing energy in from food and energy out from exercise. If exercise didn't keep the weight off, then maybe a bigger dose of exercise was needed.

The American College of Sports Medicine highlighted this issue of exercise dose in its 2009 position statement on physical activity for weight maintenance, stating that the amount of physical activity needed for weight maintenance after weight loss is uncertain. Moreover, it stated that there is a lack of randomised controlled trials in this area that use state-of-the-art techniques to monitor the energy balance of participants.

Fortunately, some of the authors of the position statement went on to use state-of-the-art techniques to monitor energy balance in their own randomised controlled trial. In 2015, they enrolled overweight adults into a 10-month aerobic exercise program and compared the energy intake of those who lost weight with the energy intake of those who didn't lose weight while on the program. They found that those who didn't lose weight were indeed taking in more calories.

Mystery of the disappearing calories

But there's something else in that 2015 study's energy measurements that is quite interesting. By the end of the study, the number of total daily calories the exercisers burned was not significantly different from what the nonexercisers burned. And this was in spite of the fact that trainers verified the exercisers burned an extra 400 to 600 calories per session at their nearly daily exercise sessions. Why didn't those extra exercise calories show up in the total daily calories burned?

The answer to that question may help explain why exercise doesn't always help you keep the weight off: Your metabolism responds to regular exercise by decreasing the number of calories you burn when you're not exercising.

That's according to the constrained total energy expenditure hypothesis that spurred the current debate.

Researchers recently tested the hypothesis by measuring the non-exercise calorie burn of 29 obese adults over a nearly 24-hour period, both before and after a six-month exercise program. They found that the calories they burned when they weren't working out did decrease after months of regular exercise – but only in those who were prescribed the higher of two different exercise doses.

Those who exercised at the lower dose for general health, meaning they burned an extra 800 to 1,000 calories per week, saw no change in their metabolic rate. But those who exercised at the higher dose to lose weight or maintain weight loss, meaning they burned an extra 2,000 to 2,500 calories per week, had a decrease in their metabolic rate by the study's end.

Exercise for health

Perhaps both sides of the debate are right. If you want to lose a modest amount of weight, then a new exercise routine might make a modest contribution toward meeting that goal.

However, as others have said, don't fool yourself into thinking you can 'outrun a bad diet' by simply exercising more. There is a diminishing marginal return to exercise – you eventually take less weight off for the additional exercise you put in.

But even if extra exercise might not help you lose weight and keep it off, there are still the other great health dividends that regular exercise pays out.

18 July 2023

THE CONVERSATION

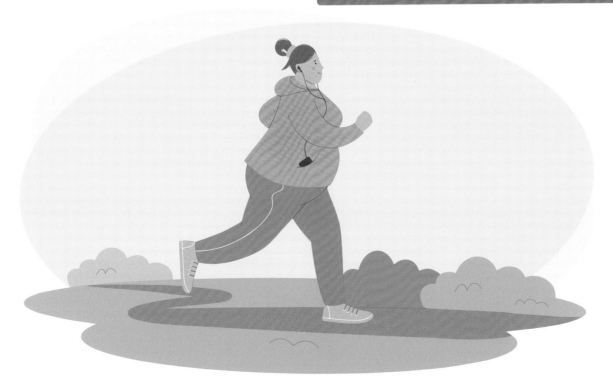

Further Reading/ Useful Websites

Useful Websites

www.bant.org.uk

www.bda.uk.com

www.cam.ac.uk

www.healtheuropa.com

www.independent.co.uk

www.inews.co.uk

www.nesta.org.uk

www.nhs.net

www.nutrition.org.uk

www.openaccessgovernment.org

www.parliament.uk

www.telegraph.co.uk

www.theconversation.com

www.theguardian.com

www.who.int

Where can I find help?

Below are some telephone numbers, email addresses and websites of agencies or charities that can offer support or advice if you, or someone you know, needs it.

Your GP
Visit your GP for advice if you have any concerns about your weight. They can refer you, if need be, to services that can help with weight management.

NHS website
www.nhs.uk/conditions/obesity

The British Association for Nutrition and Lifestyle Medicine (BANT)
www.bant.org.uk

British Dietetic Association
www.bda.uk.com

Diabetes UK
www.diabetes.org.uk

Obesity UK
www.obesityuk.org.uk

Further Reading

Pages 2-4 : Reprinted from www.who.int, Obesity and overweight, Copyright 2021, Accessed on 27/7/2023; https://www.who.int/news-room/fact-sheets/detail/obesity-and-overweight

Pages 32-36: https://bant.org.uk/the-fight-against-ultra-processed-foods-and-food-labelling-loopholes/

BMI (body mass index)

An abbreviation which stands for 'body mass index' and is used to determine whether an individual's weight is in proportion to their height. If a person's BMI is below 18.5 they are usually seen as being underweight. If a person has a BMI greater than or equal to 25, they are classed as overweight and a BMI of 30 and over is obese. As BMI is the same for both sexes and adults of all ages, it provides the most useful population-level measure of overweight and obesity. However, it should be considered a rough guide because it may not correspond to the same degree of 'fatness' in different individuals (e.g. a body builder could have a BMI of 30 but would not be obese because his weight would be primarily muscle rather than fat).

Carbohydrate

Carbohydrates (also called carbs) are a type of macronutrient found in certain foods and drinks. Sugars, starches and fibre are carbohydrates.

Diabetes

A disease in which the body's ability to produce or respond to insulin in impaired.

Diet

The variety of food and drink that someone eats on a regular basis. The phrase 'on a diet' is also often used to refer to a period of controlling what one eats while trying to lose weight.

Dietary Inequality

Where inequalities in the food system mean people in low-income groups eat less healthily than those on higher incomes.

Exercise

Physical activity that helps to improve and maintain a healthy body and mind. Exercise can be as easy as walking, swimming or dancing, to more intensive activity such as weight training, aerobics or High-Intensity Interval Training (HIIT).

Fat

Fat is an essential part of our diet. Our bodies require small amounts of `good fat` to function and help prevent disease. However, too much fat, especially the wrong type of fat, can cause serious health problems such as obesity, higher blood pressure and cholesterol levels, which in turn lead to a greater risk of heart disease. The two main types of fat are saturated and unsaturated. Unsaturated fats (e.g. found in oily fish) are generally considered better for us than saturated fats (such as dairy products, like cheese).

Fibre

Dietary fibre (sometimes called `roughage`) is the part of fruit, vegetables and wholefoods which cannot be digested by the body. It aids digestion by giving the gut bulk to squeeze against in order to move food through the digestive system. There are two types of fibre: soluble and insoluble.

Fitness

The condition of being physically healthy (e.g. described as being in shape). Remember, fitness can also apply to our mental health and well-being. A high level of fitness is usually the result of regular exercise and a proper nutrition regime.

Food poverty

When people struggle to afford food. The UK has seen an increase in the use of food banks and food parcels. The Trussel Trust food bank use remains at a record high with over one million three-day emergency food supplies given to people in crisis in 2015/16.

National Food Strategy

The National Food Strategy was introduced in England in 2020. Its intention is to ensure that the food system delivers safe, healthy, affordable food regardless of where people live or what they earn.

Nutrition

The provision of materials needed by the body for growth, maintenance and sustaining life. Commonly when people talk about nutrition, they are referring to the healthy and balanced diet we all need to eat in order for the body to function properly.

Obesity

When someone is overweight to the extent that their BMI is 30 or above, they are classed as obese. Obesity is increasing in the UK and is associated with a number of health problems, such as an increased risk of heart disease and type 2 diabetes. Worldwide obesity has more than doubled since 1980 and this is most likely due to our more sedentary lifestyle, combined with a lack of physical exercise.

Overweight

A body weight that is greater than what is considered to normal or healthy in relation to height. An overweight person BMI would be between 25 and 29.9. This does not, however, mean that an overweight person is fat – people who are muscular can have a higher BMI without much fat.

Protein

Proteins are chains of amino acids that allow the body to build and repair body tissue. Protein is found in dairy foods, meat, fish and soya beans.

Sugar

Sugar is a carbohydrate that is a naturally occurring nutrient that makes food taste sweet. There are a number of different sugars: glucose and fructose are found in fruit and vegetables; milk sugar is known as lactose; maltose (malt sugar) is found in malted drinks and beer; and sucrose comes from sugar cane or beet and is often referred to as `table` or `added` sugar. It also occurs naturally in some fruit and vegetables.

Sugar tax

Introduced in April 2018, the soft drinks industry levy (SDIL), or 'sugar tax', is a levy applied to UK-produced or imported soft drinks containing added sugar.

Index